Papal Paralysis

Papal Paralysis

How the Vatican Dealt with the AIDS Crisis

R. John Kinkel

LEXINGTON BOOKS
Lanham • Boulder • New York • Toronto • Plymouth, UK

Published by Lexington Books
A wholly owned subsidiary of Rowman & Littlefield
4501 Forbes Boulevard, Suite 200, Lanham, Maryland 20706
www.rowman.com

10 Thornbury Road, Plymouth PL6 7PP, United Kingdom

British Library Cataloguing in Publication Information Available

Library of Congress Cataloging-in-Publication Data

Kinkel, R. John.
Papal paralysis : how the Vatican dealt with the AIDS crisis / R. John Kinkel.
pages cm
Includes bibliographical references and index.
ISBN 978-0-7391-7684-9 (cloth : alk. paper)—ISBN 978-0-7391-7685-6 (electronic)
1. AIDS (Disease)—Religious aspects—Catholic Church. 2. Church work with the sick—Catholic Church. I. Title.
BX2347.8.A52K56 2014
261.8′321969792—dc23 2013036294

∞™ The paper used in this publication meets the minimum requirements of American National Standard for Information Sciences—Permanence of Paper for Printed Library Materials, ANSI/NISO Z39.48-1992.

Printed in the United States of America

To Norma, Jonathan, Danielle

Contents

Illustrations

Tables

Acknowledgments

The students who have studied medical sociology with me over the years deserve special thanks for speaking out about people who suffer and die for seemingly no good reason. Several years ago many of my undergraduate students were shocked to learn that certain religious denominations opposed the use of condoms to fight the spread of AIDS, namely, the Roman Catholic Church, Muslim groups in Malawi, and Seventh-Day Adventists in various parts of Africa. Because the Catholic Church is so large (1.2 billion members) I decided to investigate why this group was so opposed to a public health policy that seemed to be a "no-brainer" to most of my students. Hence, I began work on the book, *Papal Paralysis*, which has taken up a considerable amount of my time in the last four years.

This book is really a culmination of my life's work, which for thirty-five years has covered a long list of my sociological interests: crime, deviance, substance abuse, suicide, religion, and mental health. Never have I found a topic so intriguing as the Catholic Church's response to the AIDS crisis. The story of this tragedy has flown under the radar for the previous three decades, and now the world needs to know how papal power and authority failed to stand with those who were at risk for contracting a deadly disease.

I greatly appreciate the efforts of editors and officials at Lexington Books for believing in this research project and helping me to bring it to fruition. Eric Wrona has shown extraordinary patience when I missed deadlines and misunderstood key guidelines. Thank you for everything.

To the many readers of the manuscript, especially my wife Norma, I owe a huge debt of gratitude. Your thoughtful ideas and corrections have made the book all the more understandable to those who follow the workings of health policy, religion, and ethics. The following readers have been extremely helpful: Dale Olen, Charles Mueller, and Lance Kronzer.

As I look back to my younger years, it is clear that my mother, Miriam, has had a hand in my thinking and research focus as well. She spent her entire adult life working as a registered nurse and often told us stories about her work. Time and again we heard about people who were seriously ill and suffering tremendously. She did what she could to help them. This experience at home allowed me to see the importance of health care and the effective application of scientific insights to help people in need.

In my thirty-five years of learning and teaching sociology, I have met many strong professors who understood the discipline and passed on innumerable insights to their students. I am particularly grateful for having studied with Simon Dinitz, Leon Warshay, and Kent Schwirian. They have provided lasting lessons in sociology.

To my children, Jonathan and Danielle, I am deeply appreciative; I want to acknowledge their contribution to my understanding of social problems and how to fix them. These two lawyers have given me critical comments over the years that have improved my thinking and perspective on life. Bravo!

R. John Kinkel

Introduction

On January 22, 2005, Pope John Paul II reminded Catholics once again that the only way to fight HIV/AIDS was through abstinence and fidelity, not by using condoms.[1] Despite knowing of numerous objections to his policy both within and outside the church, the pope made it clear that there would be no change in his twenty-year-old policy against condoms. He died a few months later, presumably, with no regrets. After reviewing the state of the Catholic Church before and after Vatican II, *Papal Paralysis* traces John Paul's initial response to the AIDS crisis, his subsequent defense of his teaching on HIV/AIDS prevention, and the later transformation of the Roman Catholic Church's teaching on AIDS prevention by Benedict XVI in 2010. Why did it take so long for a modern, rational institution like the Catholic Church to develop a realistic policy to fight the spread of AIDS? The answer may surprise you.

First, we examine briefly the situation of the Catholic Church *before* AIDS. During the twenty years prior to the AIDS crisis, the Catholic Church was embroiled in a lengthy internal conflict over the morality of artificial birth control, the pill, condoms, and so on. The Second Vatican Council (1962–1965) tried to bring the church "up-to-date" after the cold war, but birth control was not on its official agenda. Three years after the council ended, Pope Paul VI promulgated the encyclical *Humanae Vitae* (1968) and declared that every contraceptive act was "intrinsically disordered,"[2] that is, immoral. This book will show that a substantial number of high ranking bishops and leading theologians voiced strong opposition to the pope's letter. Unfortunately, many social historians, scholars, and the public at large have forgotten that the pope's letter and its conclusions were highly controversial at the time and caused considerable pushback by clergy and laity alike. Fresh out of the deliberations of Vatican II, bishops from around the world knew that the path-breaking document *Dogmatic Constitution on the Church* (*Lumen Gentium*, 1964) embraced the doctrine of collegiality. The document teaches that the bishops of the world, collectively considered "the college of bishops," share responsibility for the governance and pastoral care of the church with the pope. *Lumen Gentium* states this clearly: "Together with their head, the supreme pontiff, and never apart from him, they [the college of bishops] have supreme and full authority for the universal church."[3] It was on October 30, 1963, that the council fathers voted overwhelmingly (yes = 2,148, no =336) to make collegiality a core teaching of Vatican II.[4] In 1968 many bishops felt they were not sufficiently consulted about the birth control decision and hence the negative reaction to *Humanae Vitae*.

In response to the pope's 1968 unilateral (non-collegial) decision on birth control, several bishops' conferences throughout the world suggested that married couples could use artificial birth control if they came to the conclusion that this action came from an informed Catholic conscience.[5] Life in the Catholic Church was very different some fifty years ago. Vatican II gave bishops a sense of boldness vis-à-vis the pope and his curia advisors. Collegiality is now clearly an essential feature of Catholic ecclesiology—at least on paper. The problem has been that popes in the post-Vatican II era have paid little attention to the teaching on collegiality; this would cause problems for the church down the road.

With the death of Pope Paul VI in 1978 and the election of John Paul II (John Paul I died after serving only thirty-three days in office), the direction of the Catholic Church took an about-face. The perception of the church as a society open to debate ended swiftly, and a new order of church governance began to emerge. The fifty-eight-year-old "Polish Pope" (Karol Wojtyla) as he was called by the news media came from Eastern Europe, and although he boasted about having two doctorates, his style was by no means academic. He brought a very narrow theological perspective to the chair of Peter, and it did not take long before some church leaders dubbed him the authoritarian pope.[6] He accepted without reservation the doctrine of *Humanae Vitae* and expected all clerics on the payroll to do the same. The laity were to fall in line as well. Soon he made it clear that in addition to his opposition to birth control, there would be no married priests, women could never be ordained to the priesthood, and liberation theology was out—it smacks of Marxism. He made the conservative association *Opus Dei* his personal prelature, which meant that members reported only to him. No other bishop in the world could tell the group what to do, only the pope. During his long reign as pope he canonized 483 saints—more than all the popes of the past five hundred years combined. The new regime of John Paul II seemed comfortable with its unique philosophy and management style. They were ready to face the world and all its challenges, or so they thought.

A second theme of this book centers on the AIDS crisis itself and what this disease meant for various societies throughout the world. On June 5, 1981, the Centers for Disease Control and Prevention (CDC) alerted Americans to a new and dangerous disease that baffled medical experts; later scientists would call it AIDS. All the average man on the street wanted to know was: how do we avoid it? The CDC told the public that a new virus had emerged in the United States and "the case histories suggested a 'cellular-immune dysfunction related to a common exposure' and a 'disease acquired through sexual contact.'"[7] In chapter 2 we will examine in detail how some people in the United States and elsewhere have acquired the virus that causes AIDS. Clearly, the second part of our inquiry has just become more complicated. According to social theorists Neil Fligstein and Doug McAdam, we could say that the world and the Catholic Church had experienced an "exogenous shock" in 1981 due to AIDS.[8] The next few years were spent trying to figure out the implications of this medical tsunami and how health care experts could cope with the pandemic.

Thirdly, *Papal Paralysis* examines how one organization, the Roman Catholic Church, dealt with the new disease and why its leaders could not agree with global medical authorities on an effective AIDS policy for over two-and-a-half decades. I am aware of the criticisms this study will probably face due to its topic and the no nonsense approach it brings to simplistic answers to world problems. Already Catholic scholars have reminded me and others that it is very important to understand how the church operates and that the church is very different from other organizations. That is true, and *Papal Paralysis* documents, in great detail, how the Catholic Church has been operating in the past thirty years regarding condoms and AIDS. After reading this book, people the world over can pass judgment on its findings about the Catholic Church and how it operates in a crisis situation.

It would be simplistic to say that the Catholic Church was unprepared in 1981 to deal with the enormous challenges brought about by AIDS. No country, no society, no religion knew how to respond at first. Political leaders waited for the medical experts to tell them what to do. Various theories circulated regarding the causes and cure for AIDS. Immediately some took the view that this was a "gay" disease, but these ideas were fueled by prejudice and ignorance, not science. One thing was evident, however: sex and AIDS were inextricably linked. The primary mode of HIV infection worldwide was clearly through sexual contact.[9] As we will see later on, the Vatican had views about sexuality that would limit its involvement in effective AIDS prevention programs from the very beginning.

Pope John Paul II's initial reaction to the AIDS crisis was simple: Catholics who are single should abstain from sexual relations and if married, they should be faithful to their spouse. That was it. Condoms could never be used to prevent AIDS because they are intrinsically evil—they frustrate the marital act, which must always be "open to the transmission of life."[10] Many Catholics took a deep breath and realized that the first "Slavic Pope" in the church's long history brought a very conservative agenda to Rome. The decision to make the cardinal from Krakow Catholicism's supreme leader in 1978 would set the stage for one of the greatest tragedies in Catholic Church history: the ruling that Catholics could not use condoms to prevent the spread of AIDS even though medical experts recommended such a program. Many people suffered and lost their lives following the pope's ethical directive.

It was not long, however, before the new pope's ideas were challenged. In the mid-1980s bishops from the United States, France, and other countries became tired of his simplistic answers to world problems, but no one could get him to change his theological perspective. After being shot in St. Peter's square by Ali Agca in May, 1981, and having survived his wounds, the Polish Pope became a cult figure. He even met with his would-be assassin in prison and forgave him. Many devoted Catholics felt John Paul was sent by God, and no one could stop his program to curb liberal reforms in the church. The feeling that surrounded his persona was that he was someone special. You had better listen to what he had to say. Who can forget the crowds chanting in St. Peter's square "John Paul 2, we love you"? For some twenty years theological skirmishes arose, but John Paul never gave in to his critics, never lost a battle. He died with his conservative boots on.

Not until 2010, when Pope Benedict XVI[11] opened the door for the use of condoms under certain circumstances to prevent the spread of AIDS, did the Catholic Church move away from its inflexible position that condoms were intrinsically evil. We will examine this papal U-turn in chapter 10. John Paul's successor heard the many criticisms leveled at him by the world's bishops; they called for reform and concluded that using a condom to prevent harm to another person was a higher form of morality than its opposite. To use a condom, even if one was in the process of committing an immoral act according to papal standards, was a positive choice in his hierarchy of Catholic values.

In conclusion, the story of the Catholic Church and AIDS is both remarkable and tragic. In a strong, defensive mode, the church over the years proclaimed to the world that it got it right. Artificial birth control was wrong and intrinsically evil. In taking this strong moral stand, the church unwittingly painted itself into a moral theology corner so that many Catholic bishops were unable to join the world community in a meaningful way to prevent the spread of AIDS. The reluctance of two popes to change and allow the use of condoms to prevent the spread of AIDS is what I call "papal paralysis." They could not move out of their age-old traditions to save lives. They thought that condoms were evil, and so their hands were tied. Many people, especially the poor and uneducated, died following the popes' directives. This historical case study documents how numerous church leaders called for reform and change, but the Vatican's supreme leaders had their heels dug in and would not hear of it. Some cardinals and bishops had argued that there should be a place in Catholic theology for ethical theories which maintain that condoms can be used to prevent the spread of AIDS. Through a slow and tedious process, some institutional church leaders came to the realization that mistakes were made. This story's ecclesiastical landscape is filled with heroes and villains, victims and victors. The Catholic Church has gone through its own rendition of the "dark ages" in modern times but during the process its weaknesses have been exposed; the sources of error have been identified. This book shows that the learning curve for popes and cardinals was never steep; it took them a very long time to comprehend the most elementary forms of social life.

NOTES

1. "Pope Says 'No' to Condom Use," *Chicago Tribune*, January 24, 2005, sec. A1. HIV, the "human immunodeficiency virus," is what causes AIDS (acquired immunodeficiency syndrome). HIV attacks the immune system so that the body becomes vulnerable to sickness, disease, and even death unless there is effective medical intervention.

2. Paul VI, encyclical letter *Humanae Vitae*, Vatican City, 1968: par. 14.

3. *Dogmatic Constitution on the Church* (*Lumen Gentium*), Second Vatican Council, November 21, 1964: par. 22.

4. Melissa Wilde, "How Culture Mattered at Vatican II: Collegiality Trumps Authority in the Council's Social Movement Organizations," *American Sociological Review* 69, no. 4 (2004): 576; also see John O'Malley, *What Happened at Vatican II* (Cambridge: Harvard University Press, 2008), 184.

5. Richard McCormick, "'Humanae Vitae' 25 Years Later," *America*, July 17, 1993.

6. "The Cologne Declaration," January 25, 1989, was signed by 163 theologians from Germany, Austria, and several other countries who objected to John Paul II's authoritarian style.

7. Centers for Disease Control (CDC), *Morbidity and Mortality Weekly Report* 50, no. 21 (2001): 429.

8. Neil Fligstein and Doug McAdam, "Toward a General Theory of Strategic Action Fields," *Sociological Theory* 29, no. 1 (2011): 5.

9. Anne M. Johnson, "Regular Review: Heterosexual Transmission of Human Immunodeficiency Virus," *British Medical Journal 296* (April 9, 1988): 1017–20.

10. Paul VI, *Humanae Vitae,* par. 11.

11. Benedict XVI, *Light of the World* (A Conversation with Peter Seewald), (San Francisco: Ignatius Press, 2010): 44.

1

+

The Church *before* AIDS

As I walked through the campus of Marquette University, Milwaukee, Wisconsin, on July 25, 1968, the usual mobs of nuns and priests were flocking to their classrooms. Just a few more summers and they would have their degrees. Many of us were caught off guard when we heard the morning news: "POPE BANS BIRTH CONTROL FOR CATHOLICS." I assure you that there was only one topic dominating the lunch hour conversations that day, and it wasn't Packer football. "I didn't see that one coming," a friend remarked. Others voiced tired lines from bygone days: *Roma locuta, causa finita,* that is, "Rome has spoken, the matter is ended." So the pope had finally announced his decision after years of deliberation; many roaming the corridors of Marquette University were none too pleased. I and many other priests wearing Roman collars became the target of undergraduate ridicule: "Your boy really dropped the ball on this one," a student jeered. We were automatically associated with a teaching that had vexed Catholics for years. I rushed to buy a newspaper in hopes of reading the actual text of the new encyclical. No luck and so we would have to wait a few days to find out what Paul VI actually wrote. The wonders of the Internet had not yet arrived. But there was no denying it; the news from Rome stated that Catholic teaching about artificial birth control would remain intact. If you are a Catholic and practicing artificial birth control, then you're disobeying the teachings of the church. This document would have a tremendous impact on the lives of Catholics throughout the world, and later on, spill over to influence the way popes set policy about condoms and AIDS.

THE BIRTH CONTROL COMMISSION

The history of the encyclical *Humanae Vitae* goes back to the suggestion of Cardinal Leo Josef Suenens to Pope John XXIII that he appoint a special birth control commission to look into this issue. In March 1963, the commission was established and six Catholic scholars agreed to serve on the board. The first session of the Second Vatican Council had just finished, and the pope wanted to head off any public debate on this controversial topic. The official title of the study group was the "Pontifical Commission for the Study of Population, Family, and Births."[1] One important task of this newly formed group was to prepare for the 1964 United Nations and World Health Organization conference on world population to be held in New Delhi. The new commission's general secretary, Fr. Henri de Riedmatten, O.P., came from the Roman Curia; it was his job to coordinate the work of these Catholic experts who would eventually become rather famous. In addition to reviewing global population issues, the six-member group[2] was to study the church's teaching on birth control and make recommendations to the pope. Most people simply referred to this committee as the Papal Birth Control Commission.

The 2,500 bishops meeting in Rome were reminded three times during the fall 1963 session of the council that "birth control as such was not to be debated in the council because it was being studied by the Papal Commission."[3] That reminder came a year after John XXIII officially opened the council and told all participants about "aggiornamento." It was his way of telling everyone that he wanted to bring the church up-to-date and needed the full cooperation of the bishops to do so. Easier said than done.

THE SECOND VATICAN COUNCIL

I first heard of the pope's idea for a council from a fellow high school student in 1959. He gave a speech about what he called an "Ecumenical Council" that the church was going to conduct. We had no clue what it was about or why it was needed. The seminary was chock-full of students, Mass was in Latin, and Gregorian chant sounded great. Little did we know that we were going to live through the experience of a lifetime. John O'Malley was not exaggerating when he wrote that "Pope John XXIII launched a process that would culminate in what was quite possibly the biggest meeting in the history of the world."[4]

"Pope John," as he was called by the media, was a very humane individual and loved to tell jokes. People revered the man, and he reciprocated by saying "I love all men and wish well to all." Yves Congar said it best when he wrote: "His human style was warm and friendly, Christian.

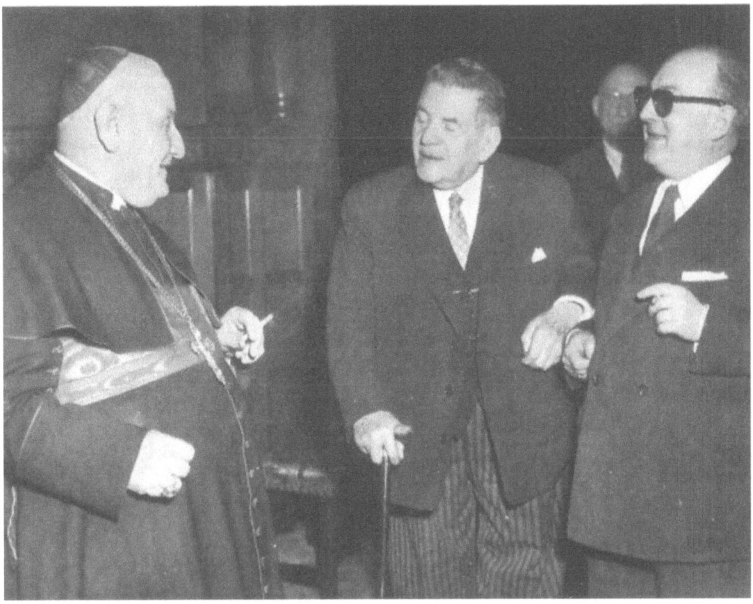

Image 1.1. The future Pope John having a smoke with guests.

Everything connected with him personally had rescued us from the horrible satrapism [barbarism] of Pius XII."[5] Pope John made it easy to forget the failings of the previous regime. One of my relatives was not a practicing Catholic in the 1960s, but due to the good humor and charity of John XXIII she came back to the church.

During the next six years we would learn from major newspapers, magazines, and books that the church was going through a period of tremendous change. All Catholics would be affected. As the years passed and we began our graduate program in theology, our brothers and sisters told us about the need for change in the church's birth control legislation. The church was way behind, they said. We would tell them the pope was working on that issue and was going to make an announcement soon. We became little experts about change in the church, and our families depended on us to keep them informed. Most of the time we did not know what was going on.

For example, the existence of the papal birth control commission was kept secret until Paul VI announced its purpose and mission in June 1963; he never disclosed who was on the commission at that time. Soon after John XXIII's death, the new pope embraced the goals of the council and the deliberations moved forward. In the fall of 1964, the council began its third session, and while debating the merits of the document on marriage and the family (*Church in the Modern World*), Cardinal John

Heenan decided to give a speech defending the doctrine of *Casti Connubii* (1930) wherein Pope Pius XI condemned birth control as intrinsically evil and immoral. Heenan wanted that teaching clearly stated in the document regarding marriage and the family. He was ignoring the order not to discuss or debate the issue of birth control, but during the council we learned that bishops don't always follow papal instructions consistently.[6] Then followed a series of four speeches that could only be described as major episcopal misgivings about the church's traditional stand on contraception.

Cardinal Emile Léger, archbishop of Montreal, observed that married couples faced many hardships in raising a family in the modern world, and he wanted to support them in any way he could. He confided to his fellow bishops that the fear of conjugal love has long paralyzed Catholic theological discussions. He told them, "We must affirm that the intimate union of the couple finds its legitimate end in itself, even when it is not directed toward procreation."[7]

Cardinal Leo Joseph Suenens followed with a speech warning about Manichean tendencies in Catholic Church teachings and that this heresy, which is characterized by hostility to the flesh as well as sexual relations, must be avoided by council fathers. He also told fellow bishops that the council should look into the possibility of working with the papal birth control commission so as to produce a comprehensive statement about marriage in the modern world. That suggestion was rejected immediately by Paul VI because he apparently wanted to have the final say on the matter after his special commission finished its deliberations. This was probably one of the biggest mistakes made during Vatican II because it appeared that the majority of the council fathers wanted an open discussion about birth control and maybe even change the church's position on it. But the pope did not give them a chance to debate and vote on the matter. The pope in conjunction with the college of bishops should have decided the issue, but the opportunity slipped through their hands as conservative forces took control.

The next speaker, Maximos IV Saigh, patriarch of Antioch, picked up on the theme of marital stress and talked about birth regulation. Maximos IV acknowledged that there was a conflict between the official doctrine of the church on birth control and the contrary practice of the vast majority of Catholic couples. "The faithful," he said, "find themselves forced to live in conflict with the law of the church, far from the sacraments, in constant anguish, unable to find a viable solution. . . . The council must find a practical solution."[8] Like Suenens, he warned the council fathers against Manichean thinking that only tolerates the activities of the flesh for the purpose of giving birth to children.

The fourth speech in this series was delivered by Cardinal Bernard Alfrink of Holland. He hammered away at the previous themes but pointed out the anxieties of loyal, married couples and the concerns Catholic families have about the number of children they can reasonably feed, clothe, and educate given the economic constraints that exist in today's world. His question to the bishops was simply this: can we bind the consciences of the faithful regarding the doctrine of *Casti Connubii* if many married couples, medical scientists, and theologians have serious doubts about its contemporary application? What is the true content of the divine law that binds the consciences of the faithful in this matter?

In reviewing the general content of these four speeches, one would assume that all these high ranking members of the clergy knew they were out of order. They were explicitly told not to discuss the issue of contraception and birth control on the council floor. But not all agreed with Vatican officials and the pope on the rules laid down on how to run a council. Robert McClory notes that the "thunderous applause that followed each of these talks showed that the ideas had resonated with many bishops."[9] But one of the council fathers was not impressed; Cardinal Alfredo Ottaviani rose from his chair the following day and declared that he was "not pleased with the statement of the text that married couples can determine the number of children they are to have. This is unheard of, from previous centuries up to our own times."[10] As we will see later on, this would not be the end of the birth control discussion at Vatican II. In short, we find that four influential council members tried to articulate the concerns and anxieties of Catholic married couples. Their efforts were not enough to sway a small group of conservative Vatican officials to rethink the norms of *Casti Connubii* which so divided the church in the 1960s. The change these speeches envisioned was not going to come easily.

There is little doubt that the teachings of Pius XI in his encyclical *Casti Connubii* were a major bone of contention for council fathers. Some felt they should be loyal to the teachings of previous popes; others questioned the legitimacy of a mandate arising during an era of political and religious extremism. Did the pope get caught up in the *Zeitgeist* of post-war Europe and lose sight of the age-old dictum of Christian thinkers—*in medio stat virtus*, that is, in the middle stands virtue? During the 1930s leaders in the Catholic Church watched the Nazi uprising in Germany as well as the popularity of Fascist dictators like Mussolini (Italy) and Franco (Spain). Those secular leaders presented the "strong man" ideology to combat European woes and not surprisingly Sophie McGrath calls this period the "age of dictators."[11] Pius XI and his theological ideas fit in nicely with this cultural trend. This was a period in history when governments reverted to extreme measures to impose their will on suspected deviants. The church would do the same. Across the pond a group of radical Christian fundamentalists hijacked the collective mind of American politicians and demanded the law of prohibition (Eighteenth Amendment). These true believers would have trashed the wedding feast at Cana (John 2:1–11). The prohibition movement emphasized that societal problems could be resolved by getting rid of alcohol. From 1920 to 1933 the United States was theoretically "dry," but the illegal production and sale of alcohol could not be stopped. The Twenty-First Amendment put an end to prohibition in 1933 when moderating forces helped the country come to its senses. Nevertheless the whole experience in Europe and the United States after World War I demonstrated that groups of dedicated ideologues can take over the reasonable tendencies of ordinary citizens as well as the basic principles of social order. With a void in regional leadership, reactionary groups can wreak havoc on the common good. The church's teachings in *Casti Connubii* (1930) must be seen in the social historical context of extremism for several reasons.

First, Pius XI was looking for ways to assert his authority on the world stage because of the long-standing "Roman Question." He negotiated with Mussolini and signed the Lateran Treaty (1929), which recognized Vatican City as an independent and neutral state. The pope was indemnified for the loss of the Papal States, and he no longer called himself the prisoner of the Vatican. But he was not really pleased with the new arrangement. Second, he signed a concordat with Hitler in 1933 in hopes that the Catholic Church could operate free from Nazi interference and oppression. The Führer had no intention of honoring that agreement. But the pope felt he had no choice and rolled his theological dice. J. N. D. Kelly reminds us of the personal flaws of Pius XI when he writes, "Armed with a strong sense of personal authority, he preferred to delegate as little as possible, and greatly reduced the role of the Sacred College."[12] Bishops became regional branch managers like they are in 2013. He came to his senses in 1937 and condemned Hitler and the Nazi regime for its anti-Catholic policies.[13] Mistakes plagued his papacy and the concordat of 1933, negotiated by Cardinal Eugenio Pacelli, was dead in the water as World War II approached. Pius XI did not respond to the famous letter sent to him by Edith Stein in 1933; she warned him about the dangers of Nazi anti-Semitism and Hitler's lust for power. Stein was a recent convert from Judaism and had subsequently joined the Carmelite sisters of Cologne. The convert-nun never heard from the pope and, like many others, died in a Nazi concentration camp; she was canonized a saint in 1998.

Pius XI's main organizational flaw was that he rarely consulted with his brother bishops on church matters and more often than not, got lost in the complicated world of foreign affairs. When the Anglican Church met for the Lambeth Conference in 1930 and approved the use of artificial birth control for its members, the pope of the depression years condemned his Protestant brothers for failing to adhere to the obvious laws of nature. Soon after he promulgated *Casti Connubii* and thereby joined a long line of dictators of that era. Thus, the letter that condemned birth control was less of a true theological statement about Christian marriage than a product of cultural extremism and papal bluster. It is not surprising that the bishops of Vatican II wondered if a new age of enlightenment should replace the philosophical and theological excesses of the 1930s. Suenens, Maximos, Alfrink, and Léger found out that the prohibition against birth control would be a lot harder to overturn than the Eighteenth Amendment of the U.S. Constitution.

Pope Paul VI supported the idea of a birth control commission after he took office in 1963 but wanted to reserve the final decision about Catholics and contraception to himself. Pius XI and Pius XII had made important statements condemning artificial birth control in the past, and perhaps Paul felt this was a papal responsibility. Given the kind of progressive proposals and decisions made by the council as well as the new theological insights contained in Vatican II's many documents, numerous priests and married couples felt there would be a change in the birth control ban. Why not? Many prominent cardinals and bishops seemed inclined to go in that direction.

The council moved forward with its crowded agenda in 1964, and soon it became clear that 1965 would see its final session. A great deal of work needed to be accomplished before the close of Vatican II, especially on documents related to religious freedom and Jewish-Christian relations. However, some of the most controversial decisions would have to be made two weeks before December 8, 1965, when the four years of meetings would officially end. Pope Paul VI apparently acquiesced to the pressure of conservatives (Cardinal Ottaviani, Fr. John Ford, and others) and informed the mixed commission working on the final draft of *Gaudium et Spes* (Church in the Modern World) that a number of changes would have to be made. On November 24, 1965, Cardinal Ottaviani read a letter to the commission written by Cardinal Amleto Cicognani, Vatican secretary of state, stating that Paul VI wanted to make several additions to the marriage and family section of *Gaudium et Spes*. The document must state that the principal end of marriage is procreation. The chapter must refer to the importance of the teachings of Pius XI and Pius XII, who condemned artificial birth control. Moreover, according to Cicognani, the pope said he wanted the council document to ban all types of contraception. That was a strange turn of events since such action would have put the birth control commission out of business. The group had not made any recommendations to the pope as yet. This last minute attempt by clerics who were unhappy with the

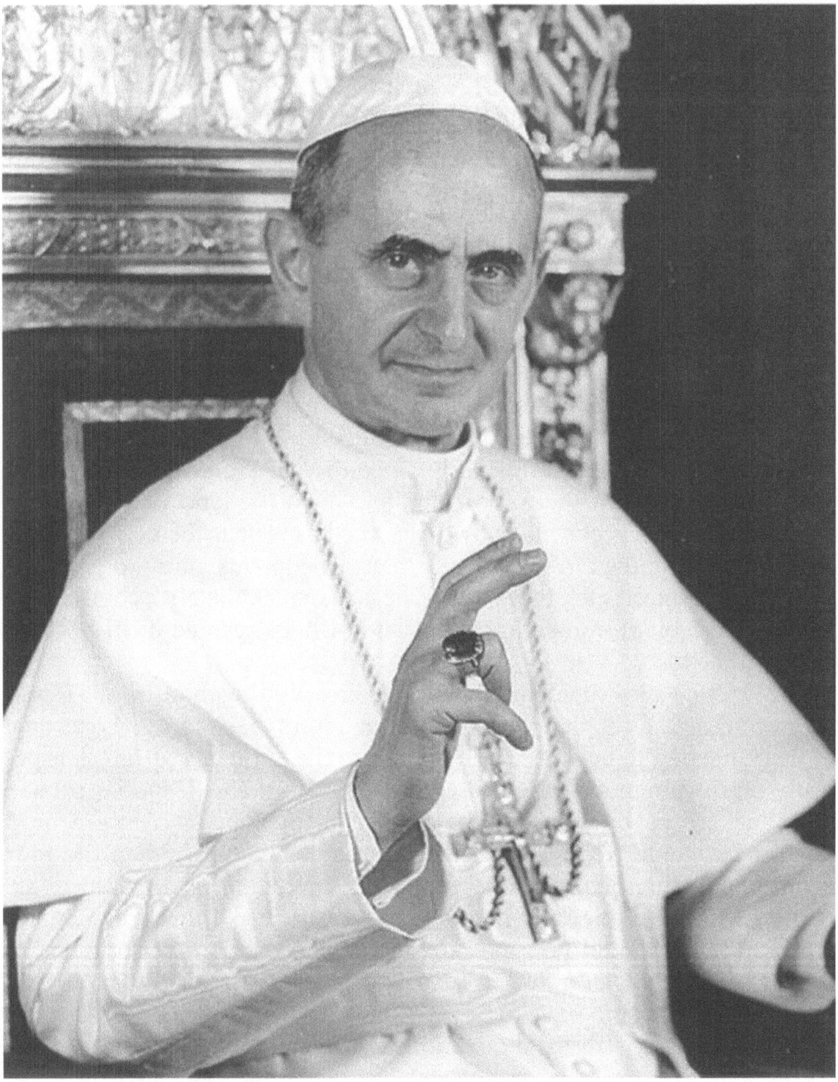

Image 1.2. Pope Paul VI continued the council after the death of Pope John in 1963.

council's actions looked promising for conservatives at first. Apparently, the pope let them have their day in court. They claimed that the pope was on their side, but would this strategy halt the forces of change?

The next day, November 25, Archbishop John Dearden of Detroit informed the mixed commission members that he objected to being "bulldozed" by disgruntled curia officials into changing the council text, which had been voted on already and approved by the world's Catholic bishops.[14] Such action was barred by council rules, he claimed. Thus Dearden led a group which approved some modifications to the council text but made sure all conservative suggestions were "rendered essentially toothless."[15] The diary of famous council peritus Yves Congar records events in a similar fashion, namely, that the pope's suggestions were accepted but utilized in "such a way that they said nothing."[16] These were the days when bishops took their jobs seriously and were not intimidated by curial officials. The last minute attempt by a small group of Vatican insiders to overturn council rules and change the sense of the approved council text was blocked. The logic used by council officials like Dearden in response to the conservatives' intervention was simple: you told us not to discuss birth control at the council; it is off the table. In a not so subtle way they were telling the pope that they would say as little as possible about birth control and let the papal commission complete its task.

POST-VATICAN II

One should remember these last-minute attempts to preserve church "orthodoxy" because the same strategy would be used with the birth control commission in 1966 with totally different results. The number of people appointed to serve on the birth control commission grew over the years (1963–1966). When it came time for members to vote on key items for the final report, there were seventy-nine Catholics serving on this advisory group, including seven cardinals and eight bishops.[17] The final voting (see table 1.1) showed that the vast majority of the commission members (87 percent) favored a change in the church's birth control teaching.

The vote was not even close. In a desperate last-minute move, Paul VI appointed Cardinal Ottaviani to the birth control commission before the 1966 final vote, even though he had never attended any of its previous meetings. In 1965 several from the American delegation suggested that the following scholars be added to the commission, but none of them were ever named to it: Yves Congar, Hans Küng, Karl Rahner, John

Table 1.1. The key commission vote: "Is contraception intrinsically evil?"

	Bishops	*non-Bishops*	*%*
No	9	60	87.3
Yes	3	4	12.7
Abstain	3	—	—
Totals	15	64	N = 79

Source: Robert McClory, *Turning Point* (New York: Crossroad, 1995), 127; Stephen Mumford (1995).

Courtney Murray, and Robert Drinan. Ottaviani was one of the seven cardinals allowed to vote on the final report, and he certainly voted against the plan for change developed over the previous four years of discussion.[18] According to Vatican protocol at the time, only the votes cast by bishops and cardinals were counted when recommendations were forwarded to the pope for study and action. The laity and lowly priests had no active voice, but we know how their votes were cast.[19] Despite these unusual quirks in the Vatican's system of counting votes, it was obvious that only three of fifteen bishops (20 percent) gave an affirmative response to the fundamental question of the day ("Is contraception intrinsically evil?"). A paltry four of sixty-four (6 percent) of the non-bishops agreed with the idea that contraception was intrinsically evil. Reform had clearly carried the day, and what is not intrinsically evil can be changed. This was considered the most important vote to be taken at the meeting, and the core reason most members asked for a new birth control policy. If contraception is not intrinsically evil, then the teaching on birth control can be reformed. When all the votes were tallied, almost 90 percent of the commission members opposed the notion that contraception was intrinsically evil. They had rejected the fundamental doctrine of *Casti Connubii.* The pope asked them to perform a task for the church, and they did it.

As is evident from table 1.1 above, the majority of bishops and cardinals cleared the way for a change in the church's birth control policy. The three opposition votes came from Ottaviani and two other conservative clerics: Morris and Colombo. The bishops/cardinals also voted on the following question: "Is contraception, as defined by the majority report, in basic continuity with tradition and the declarations of the magisterium?" The results were nine "yes" and five "no," with one abstention. To complete the day's business "the majority of the bishops and cardinals gave their formal assent to the Majority report."[20] In light of these data I find the remarks of Richard Fehring, SJ, troubling to say the least. He writes that "because there was no consensus among the members of the commission, a majority report and a minority report were eventually presented to Paul VI."[21] This is an incredible distortion of historical reality. A minority report emerged because a disgruntled set of clerics were upset because after four years of deliberation, the vast majority favored a change and the conservatives did not like it. In my view there was a clear, unequivocal message sent to the pope by his commission: drop the ban on artificial birth control. That was the consensus view of the pope's commission. The pope ignored the recommendation of loyal Catholics working for the church and decided to follow a different path.

After the vote was taken, the general secretary of the commission, Fr. Henri de Riedmatten and Cardinal Julius Doepfner, archbishop of Munich, hand-delivered the final report to the pope. According to Gerald

Slevin[22] the document strongly recommended that the church's ban on all forms of artificial birth control be lifted. In 1967 the final commission report was leaked to the press and subsequently published in the *National Catholic Reporter*, Kansas City, Missouri. All the world was now aware that the pope's four-year study commission on birth control had recommended a change and it was a drastic shift from the norms of *Casti Connubii*. Paul VI was furious that someone would leak the confidential report to the press. Now, what would he do?

Behind the scenes Cardinal Alfredo Ottaviani, prefect of the Congregation for the Doctrine of the Faith (formerly called the "Holy Office"), thought the church was about to make a grave theological error. He summoned several of his conservative allies with one goal in mind: write an "alternative" report and ask the pope to reject the commission's recommendations and findings.

With the help of fellow conservatives Fr. John Ford and Germain Grisez, both from the United States, Ottaviani crafted a position paper arguing that the pope must not change the church's teaching on birth control. On the contrary, he should maintain the doctrine enunciated in *Casti Connubii* (1930) and ban all use of contraceptives. Within weeks the aging cardinal delivered his report to Pope Paul VI. The pontiff now had two proposals on his desk: one to allow birth control and the other not to allow birth control. Which one shall it be? The Hamlet comparison is apropos: "To be or not to be: that is the question." Unlike many of Ottaviani's arguments that had been dismissed by council fathers as out of touch with mainstream Catholic theology, the pope listened intently to the senior cardinal, who felt it was his duty to defend the Catholic Church against false prophets. His cardinal coat of arms read "*semper idem*," that is, always the same. The pope was very familiar with the ideology of Alfredo Ottaviani and his behavior at the council (see table 1.2). Paul VI must have seen something compelling in this stalwart apostle of right-wing Catholicism who was going blind after almost fifty years of service to the church since his priestly ordination.

Table 1.2. Cardinal Ottaviani at the Vatican Council.

1. He opposed liturgical renewal: advocated keeping the Mass in Latin.
2. He led the charge against the concept of collegiality.
3. He objected to the document on religious liberty and separation of church and state.
4. He boycotted the council for two weeks because of an unfavorable response by bishops to one of his interventions.
5. He threatened to leave the council if he did not receive an apology from Cardinal Frings who had called for curia reform.
6. He opposed the idea of calling a council in the first place.

Source: John O'Malley, *What Happened at Vatican II*, 138, 192, 193, 213.

The pope knew that the majority of the bishops at Vatican II had a negative opinion of him. For example, on November 8, 1963, Ottaviani scolded council moderators for not submitting issues related to collegiality to his Doctrinal Commission so its members could review them. His intervention "angered many bishops to the point of talking, in private, about his removal as president of his commission. Members of the commission itself sent Paul VI a petition to replace Ottaviani, but no action was taken on it."[23] The pope tolerated the conservative approach of this curial cardinal and later embraced the principles of Pius XI in his 1968 encyclical.

Paul VI knew what Ottaviani stood for, and it was pure conservative theology—the kind of perspective rejected by council fathers. The cardinal opposed all the key changes the council majority had passed overwhelmingly. He even opposed John XXIII when the pope called the council in the first place. Little wonder why Pope John once called Ottaviani "a child."[24] When he failed to get key statements included in the chapter on marriage (*Gaudium et spes*), he wrote this note to the pope: "I did all possible to have the Commission accept the modifications of Your Holiness, but was always in the minority."[25] Compromise? Never. The man always felt he was right, even when his fellow colleagues refused to accept his unconvincing arguments. Ottaviani's approach throughout the council was to "shut down" opposition bishops and theologians; they were wrong and he was right. Cardinal Franz Konig makes this rather telling observation:

> I had already got to know Cardinal Ottaviani, the head of the Holy Office, as the Congregation for the Doctrine of the Faith was still called then, under Pope Pius XII. I remember bumping into him once, soon after Pius XII first allowed evening Masses. He came up to me and said, "What do you say? One can now celebrate Mass in the evening. Don't people laugh when you announce an evening Mass?" It took me a little time to see what he meant, but it was a typical Ottaviani reaction. There is a fixed order of things which must never be changed—*Semper idem* was after all his motto. As change was inconceivable to him, it seemed also in a strange way ludicrous.[26]

If Ottaviani had his way during the council, the Mass would still be in Latin, collegiality would be relegated to the dust bin of church history, and communion under both forms a pious dream. Ironically it was to this man, who could not get council fathers to subscribe to his views on liturgy, collegiality, or church-world politics, that the pope turned for advice on the birth control matter. The curial cardinal gave him the answer he was looking for: *semper idem*. Roman Catholics would pay a price and so would the credibility of the church's teaching authority.

Many argue that Pope Paul should have seen Ottaviani's character flaws for what they were and forced him to retire after his inauspicious behavior at the council. Cardinal Suenens said as much at the end of the council, but the pope could not bear to fire his old curia friend. Paul VI had worked in the Roman Curia for twenty-five years before becoming the archbishop of Milan and learned to "live and let live." That was a crucial mistake unless one takes the position that Paul VI was using him to promote his latent conservative ideology on marriage. It appears from observations made at the council that Ottaviani could no longer objectively study a theological problem and come up with a realistic solution. What was his problem? Two explanations come to mind.

First, it is obvious that he was one of the most disliked bishops at the council. Council fathers even made him the butt of their jokes. Example: One morning Cardinal Ottaviani hailed a cab and told the driver, "Take me to the council." Immediately, the cabbie headed for Trent.[27]

Why did he act in such a way that so many of his fellow bishops concluded that he was a pure ideologue? How could such a person be placed in a position of authority and manage church affairs during a period of great historical importance? A recent study of pathological altruism (PA) by Barbara Oakley and associates may give us some insights into this man's career path and actions.[28] PA is a disorder characterized by any behavior or personal tendency wherein the stated aim of the person with the disorder is to promote the welfare of another. That sounds good, but instead of achieving beneficial outcomes for another person, the so-called altruistic person's behavior leads to substantial negative consequences for the victim. Think of the famous Ronald Reagan quip about the man who comes to your front door and says, "I'm from the government and I am here to help." That's pretty altruistic, but will you be better off after opening the door to this stranger? For Ottaviani it was always, "I am from the Vatican and want to help. I am from the Holy Office and want you to stop talking that way. I want to help you understand what the true Catholic position is on this. I want to help you get over this." The helping of another was really a judgment against the person and the offering of corrective measures. In the end this is a not-so-subtle case of self-promotion. That's what pathological altruism is all about. PA sufferers want other people to think they are being served. Bishops at the Second Vatican Council caught on to this clerical con game right away. Paul VI apparently did not.

A second reason people found Ottaviani so disconnected from many of his colleagues can be found by reviewing the work of Mark Blais, Massachusetts General Hospital.[29] Here we find a rich treasure trove of research about people like the cardinal everyone loved to hate. It does not take a lot of work to see that Ottaviani was probably suffering from narcissistic personality disorder.[30] He exhibited all the key components: (1) There is grandiose thinking from the outset; "My ideas are right, I must save the church from error." (2) Preoccupation with power to preserve the status quo. It is obvious when studying his moves at the council and later on with the birth control commission that change was inconceivable to him. He sought high positions in the church to control underlings and the pope himself. That will make his ideas dominate every time. (3) Lack of empathy toward others. He was not sensitive to other peoples' line of thinking—just to correct their thinking. He was arrogant and contemptuous of the opposition.

As a member of the curia in the 1950s, he was responsible for sanctions leveled against Yves Congar, Karl Rahner, and John Courtney Murray—theologians whom council fathers depended on during Vatican II to bring "aggiornamento" to the church.[31] Their ideas were legitimized by council fathers whereas Ottaviani's were by and large rejected. What has been mistakenly viewed as an old man's odd and eccentric ways ought to be seen in their true light. The pope and other Vatican officials were apparently unaware that a very disturbed and troubled person was living among them with the daily objective of leading the church along the lines dictated by personal needs and compulsions, not church growth and development. Under the guise of fidelity to the teachings of previous popes, he was really responding to his own psychological flaws that had little or nothing to do with advancing Christian belief in the contemporary world. Some looked at him as an old war horse who could not give up; he wanted to beat down the forces for change, which he saw as a threat to church orthodoxy. But there was more to it than that. A man who was significantly impaired had a major role in crafting a birth control policy that the vast majority of Catholics working on the pope's commission concluded was inadequate and a relic of the past. Would an unpopular Italian cleric be able to overcome the governing principles laid down by Augustine and the Council of Carthage—the concept of one man, one vote? Yes, because the rules of Augustine were clearly not the Ottaviani way.

Some scholars depict Pope Paul as "Hamlet-like," and that he was; papal insiders felt he was always weighing the pros and cons of various decisions he had to make. But it would be a mistake to think of him as an impartial observer, examining all aspects of a proposal and then coming down on the side of the meritorious theological argument. When it came down to the bottom line, he seemed to be a closet conservative when dealing with church views on sexual morality. But on social justice issues he was a progressive along the lines of *Rerum Novarum,* 1891 (need for social justice) and *Pacem in Terris,* 1963 (respect for human rights, common good)—two of the greatest social justice documents ever crafted by officials in the Roman Catholic Church. Paul VI's visit to the UN in 1965 and his famous speech there, together with his encyclical *Populorum Progressio,* put him on the "liberal" side of the scale measuring social reform, justice, and peace. He was a complex individual with positive and negative features. He fought the good fight, but lost the war against Catholic sexual extremism.

ENTER *HUMANAE VITAE*

Without doubt birth control was one of the biggest decisions Pope Paul had to make during his papacy. Within a year of the papal commission's final report, the broad outlines of the encyclical *Humanae Vitae* had begun to take shape. Cardinal Giovanni Montini became the first modern pope elected during a council and always had a group of liberals and conservatives to test the waters of decision making. "Should I approve this?" "What does the majority of the council think?" Yes, he was Hamlet-like. Alone with the curia and the domineering presence of Ottaviani, the pope decided in favor of the status quo. The work of the birth control commission and its conclusions would be scuttled in favor of an insider position paper that argued for no change. He never wrote another encyclical after *Humanae Vitae* (1968), but he did send out numerous apostolic letters before he died ten years later. In contrast, John Paul II wrote an encyclical almost every year during his first ten years in office. Paul VI was shell-shocked by the world's reaction to his views on birth control. He completely misread the signs of the times. That was rather easy to do when depending on the insights of Ottaviani.

For almost forty years scholars have asked church historians this simple set of questions. What if the bishops attending Vatican II would have taken up the birth control issue as Suenens had suggested in 1964 and included their findings in the document *The Church in the Modern World*? Or, what if the pope would have followed the recommendations of the papal birth control commission and agreed that change was the right path to follow? That would have made the condoms/AIDS controversy irrelevant during the next decade. In my view there was a clear, unequivocal message sent to the pope by his commission: drop the ban on artificial birth control. The pope just refused to follow the recommendations of a large and dedicated staff of good, educated Roman Catholics.

A small but powerful group ensconced in the Vatican bureaucracy had their way. Their norms became doctrine through *Humanae Vitae*. In the late 1960s this ruling was severely criticized because it failed to take into account the needs of young families and the importance of sexual intimacy for a meaningful married life. The commission was well versed regarding the Crowley survey of Catholic married couples, which demonstrated that the natural family planning method (rhythm) had many negative side effects and caused harm to numerous Catholic marriages.[32] The one birth control method the church approved of did not work for the majority of Catholic families.

Bishops' conferences around the world gave the new encyclical mixed reviews. Certainly, some bishops and priests spoke in favor of the pope's decision, but a significant number of journalists and scholars pointed out that *Humanae Vitae's* publication marked the first time in the twentieth century that there was open, large-scale dissent by priests and bishops regarding an important papal teaching. We are not even talking here about the laity's response.

The "Winnipeg Statement," crafted by the Canadian bishops, is a case in point. The pope's letter brought the church to an "hour of crisis," the bishops wrote, and they reminded those who could not accept the teachings of the new encyclical that they were not "shut off from the body of the faithful."[33] Some segments of the church fell in line and supported the pope, at least in public. The Dutch bishops stressed the importance of an informed individual conscience when dealing with birth control, and this turned out to be the position of the German hierarchy as well. The U.S. bishops issued their response to *Humanae Vitae* in November 1968, and their pastoral letter included the norms of licit dissent from church doctrine. In any case, they warned Catholics that they may never question the teaching authority of the church.[34] The bishops' statement went on to say that individuals can in good conscience use contraceptives if they have made an honest attempt to accept and follow the teaching of *Humanae Vitae* but simply could not.

Cardinal Suenens took a different approach to the pope's letter. He objected to the way Paul VI arrived at the birth control decision, that is, he did not follow the council's norms of collegiality. The pope decided an important ethical and moral question without consulting the full body of the bishops. Instead of following the recommendations of the papal birth control commission, he allowed the curia to take over and make the decision. The cardinal probably had a point. Pius IX in 1854 asked Catholic bishops their opinion before proclaiming the dogma of the Immaculate Conception. The pope wanted to assert as dogma that the Blessed Virgin Mary, from the moment of her conception, was preserved from all stain of original sin. The pope's survey of 603 bishops revealed that 546 responded in the affirmative. The dogma was proclaimed on December 8, 1854. Likewise, Pius XII asked bishops their views before he defined the assumption of the Blessed Virgin Mary as a dogma of faith in 1950. Paul VI decided to go it alone on this one, with Ottaviani pressuring him at every step of the way.

Bishops and cardinals have spoken bluntly at times regarding papal pronouncements and not incurred many sanctions. When priests do the same, however, it is another story. The case of Fr. Charles Curran, theology professor at Catholic University of America, illustrates what happens to clerics who do not agree with Vatican directives, no matter how its norms are proclaimed. Not long after the publication of the new encyclical, Curran publicly dissented from the church's ban on artificial birth control and issued a major theological statement about it. Curran objected to the basic thrust of Pope Paul's teaching and asserted "spouses may responsibly decide according to their conscience that artificial contraception in some circumstances is permissible and indeed necessary to preserve and foster the value and sacredness of marriage."[35] About six hundred theologians and scholars, including preeminent moral theology professor Fr. Bernard Häring signed the Curran statement. After some ten years of feuding, the university attempted to fire Curran for his actions, but he was not barred from teaching there until 1986. He finally left the university in 1988. One should note that it was not Paul VI who pulled the plug on Fr. Curran, but rather the regime of John Paul II that cracked down on Curran and other theologians who did not uphold "Catholic doctrine." Academic freedom at a Catholic university has its limits.

The case of Hans Küng (council peritus) and the German church is illustrative of the "laissez faire" approach of Paul VI to dissent. In a letter to the Congress of German Catholics, Pope Paul wrote: "May the lively debate aroused by our encyclical lead to a better knowledge of God's will."[36] Although Küng made it clear that he had serious doubts about the major conclusions of *Humanae Vitae,* he had bigger fish to fry. His book, *Infallible? An Inquiry* (1970), shook the Holy See's frescoed halls and ceilings by opening a debate regarding the very nature and scope of papal power. After nine years of conflict with the Vatican over his central thesis that the doctrine of infallibility needed to be refined and reexamined, Küng was removed from his chair as professor of Catholic theology at the University of Tübingen, Baden-Württemberg, Germany. Here again we see that John Paul had a very different approach on how to deal with church conflict than did Paul VI. The Polish Pope had Küng fired one year after he took office in 1978; Paul VI did not even sanction the German theologian. Throughout the post-Vatican II period, Rome was quite tolerant of diversity and felt debate had a place in Catholic Church theology, given the teachings of the council regarding the importance of conscience and religious freedom. But John Paul II ushered in a new era of thinking toward those who disagreed with what he called official church teaching: they had to be silenced. They did not represent true Catholic doctrine. With the election of John Paul II, the Catholic Church was given a charismatic leader who had his own opinions on how the church should be run. He consulted with a narrow group of clerics who agreed with his general principles. A new era of Catholic leadership arrived from Poland and for all practical purposes it was "my way or the highway." The Polish Pope's program would not be a useful approach in dealing with a future world problem, the AIDS pandemic. The issue of papal paralysis had its roots in the era of Vatican II, and it emerged in full force during the condoms/ AIDS controversy—the central theme of this book.

CONCLUSION

After a review of modern Catholic birth control teaching, one is inclined to ask: why is the United States embroiled in another cantankerous debate with the Catholic Church about birth control in 2013? Isn't this really old news? Apparently not. This topic never seems to go away—condoms and AIDS, birth control and religious freedom. When will it all end? U.S. Catholic Church officials have challenged a federal mandate that would require employer-provided health insurance to pay for, among other things, an employee's birth control program.[37] Catholic bishops administer numerous organizations in their dioceses, and they argue that forcing them to provide health care that includes birth control would violate their religious freedom. Many people in this debate ask: has the Catholic Church ever demonstrated that this particular religious norm is so central to its religious teachings that it should be honored by secular legislative action? Do Catholics claim this as a core belief? Doubts arise when one examines the facts in the case.

1. The basis for the Catholic norm of "no contraception" arose primarily because of Pius XI's 1930 letter, *Casti Connubii*, which condemned all artificial birth control as immoral. Vatican II conservatives like Ottaviani maintained that such doctrine was irreformable. We should recall that this teaching of Pius XI arose during a period of political and philosophical extremism wherein church leaders (the pope) followed the cultural tendency to overreact to social problems and assert principles that have limited validity in post-war Western civilization. The leaders of that era dictated policy and the simple, uneducated people were to follow orders. Pius XI foolishly signed a concordat with Hitler in 1933 hoping Catholics would be spared Nazi persecution and then four years later said he made a mistake and condemned the Führer. He did not heed the warnings of Edith Stein—now a saint—who wrote a famous letter to the pope asking him to condemn Nazi anti-Semitism. The seriously flawed public policies of this pope must be juxtaposed against his radical, uncompromising stand on contraception. He liked to work alone and did not consult with

others very much. Vatican II bishops (1962–1965) wanted to revisit the 1930s teachings of Pius XI but were blocked by Pope Paul VI.

2. John XXIII set up a birth control commission to study this problem in 1963, since he knew Catholics had a problem with *Casti Connubii*. When this group of Catholic experts met and decided to recommend major changes to the pope, Paul VI rejected their overwhelming call to lift the ban on artificial birth control. He instead sided with the conservative cardinal Ottaviani, whom council fathers considered out of touch with church pastoral experience. The cardinal was smarting after most of his proposals were rejected by council fathers and hoped for a face-saving victory in the birth control debate. That would be a huge face-saving device. Fearing a palace (curia) revolt, Paul VI promulgated his encyclical *Humanae Vitae* (1968), which banned birth control; the letter was not received well by the laity and a ten year debate ensued.
3. In 1978 Pope John Paul II brought his conservative Eastern European theology to Rome and made birth control a defining rule for his administration. Everyone must accept the teachings of *Humanae Vitae*. When the Polish Pope died in 2005, a Gallup poll published that year revealed that in the United States, 78 percent of all Catholics interviewed supported the concept that church members should be allowed to practice birth control. For all his efforts, John Paul did not convince Catholics that the church understood pastoral theology and the family. Throughout his almost three-decade reign as supreme pontiff and principal teacher of the church, he was unable to convince the vast majority of Catholics that he was right on the birth control issue.

Many people who review these historical facts are likely to conclude that birth control has never been properly discussed in an open church forum, and thus, members have had an unpopular and questionable teaching imposed on them by celibate men who have no experience of married life. Conservative bishops and popes set the norms, but few of the laity follow them. Without considering the historical context and underhanded tactics used by the Roman Curia to formulate Catholic family morality, U.S. lawmakers would be foolish to let Catholic Church leaders claim their religious freedom is being violated by the Affordable Care Act (2010). The whole landscape of Catholic discourse on this matter since 1930 has been riddled by violations of individual religious freedom. It is disingenuous for Catholic leaders to ask secular lawmakers to honor their religious traditions when so few believers follow the anti–birth control norm in everyday life. The United States must assert the rule of law which protects all citizens and not the rule of several popes that only 20 percent of Catholics follow. Conservative cardinals like Dolan of New York have had years to convince Catholics that their sacred norms on contraception should be followed. These efforts have failed. Bishops today should not lobby for special favors and exemptions that few Catholic families want to follow. It is a papal norm that is immoral and greatly unjust.

NOTES

1. Robert McClory, *Turning Point* (New York: Crossroad, 1995), 40.
2. The initial six members of the commission were John Marshall, Clement Mertens, Stanislas de Lestapis, Henri de Riedmatten, Pierre von Rossum, and Jacques Mertens de Wilmars.
3. John W. O'Malley, *What Happened at Vatican II* (Cambridge: Harvard University Press, 2008), 237.
4. O'Malley, *What Happened*, 18.
5. Ives Congar, *My Journal of the Council* (Collegeville, MN: Liturgical Press, 2012), 5.
6. O'Malley, *What Happened*, 6. There were three major issues that were considered so sensitive that Vatican officials withheld them from the council's agenda: clerical celibacy, birth control, and reform of the Roman Curia.
7. Quoted in McClory, *Turning Point*, 59.
8. Quoted in Robert Kaiser, *The Politics of Sex and Religion* (Kansas City, MO: Leaven Press, 1985), 65.
9. McClory, *Turning Point*, 61.
10. Quoted in Kaiser, *The Politics of Sex*, 67.
11. Sophie McGrath, "In the Age of Dictators: Edith Stein and Pope Pius XI in Conversation," *Australian eJournal of Theology* 3 (August, 2004): 1.
12. J. N. D. Kelly, *The Oxford Dictionary of Popes* (New York: Oxford University Press, 1986), 318.
13. See Pius XI famous encyclical letter *Mit Brennender Sorge*, 1937.
14. McClory, *Turning Point*, 83.
15. McClory, *Turning Point*, 84
16. Congar, *My Journal of the Council*, 855.
17. McClory, *Turning Point*, 190. He provides a list of commission members; note that Archbishop Karol Wojtyla did not attend the last meeting and thus he could not vote because communist officials in Poland would not give him permission to travel outside the country.
18. Kaiser, *The Politics of Sex*, 174; Colombo, Ottaviani, and Morris were the three negative votes.
19. Stephen Mumford, "The Vatican's Role in the World Population Crisis: The Untold Story," *Journal of Social, Political and Economic Studies* 20, no. 1 (1995): 35, www.population-security.org/phil95.htm (accessed November 5, 2012).
20. McClory, *Turning Point*, 127.
21. Richard Fehring, "An Analysis of the Majority Report," *Life and Learning XIII* (2003): 124, epublications.marquette.edu/nursing_fac/48/ (accessed June 9, 2012).

22. Gerald Slevin, "New Birth Control Commission Papers Reveal Vatican's Hand," *National Catholic Reporter*, March 23, 2011, http://ncronline.org/news/vatican/new-birth-control-commission-papers-reveal-vaticans-hand (accessed February 23, 2012).

23. O'Malley, *What Happened*, 185.

24. J. J. Scarisbrick, "An Historian's Reflections on Yves Congar's Mon Journal de Concile," in *Yves Congar: Theologian of the Church*, ed. Gabriel Flynn (Louvain: Peeters Press, 2005), 252.

25. Xavier Rynne, *The Fourth Session* (New York: Farrar, Straus and Giroux, 1966), 224.

26. Franz König, "It Must be the Holy Spirit," *The Tablet* (December 21–28, 2002): 4–6.

27. The Council of Trent convened after the Protestant Reformation and is known for its condemning actions and conservative theology, which dominated the Catholic Church for more than two centuries.

28. Barbara Oakley, Ariel Knafo, et al., eds., *Pathological Altruism* (New York: Oxford University Press, 2011), 3–9.

29. Mark Blais et al., "Personality and Personality Disorders" in Theodore Stern et al., *Massachusetts General Hospital Comprehensive Clinical Psychiatry*, 1st ed. (Philadelphia: Mosby Elsever, 2009), chapter 39.

30. William Cockerham, *Sociology of Mental Disorder*, 8th ed. (New York: Prentice Hall, 2011), 47.

31. Scarisbrick, "An Historian's," 254–59; also see O'Malley, *What Happened*, 87–88.

32. McClory, *Turning Point*, 133.

33. Canadian Conference of Catholic Bishops, "Canadian Bishops' Statement on the Encyclical *Humanae Vitae*," Ottawa, Canada, September 27, 1968.

34. Quoted in Richard McCormick, "'*Humanae Vitae*' 25 Years Later," *America*, July 17, 1993, 21.

35. McCormick, "'Humanae *Vitae*' 25 Years Later," 21–22.

36. McCormick, "'*Humanae Vitae'* 25 Years Later," 22.

37. Laurie Goodstein, "Catholics File Suits on Contraception Coverage," *New York Times*, May 21, 2012.

2

✛

AIDS Hits America

I had just parked our minivan near my son's elementary school in Grosse Pointe, Michigan. Ben came running out of the school gym toward us and looked completely out of breath. "JJ," he yelled to my son, "Magic has AIDS." They looked at each other as if to say: he's gonna die! At that time many thought AIDS was a death sentence. Magic Johnson, the star basketball player at Michigan State University and NBA champion with the L.A. Lakers had the dreaded disease; his fans were in a state of shock. He had tested positive for the HIV virus[1] that causes AIDS and soon chose to retire from professional basketball. As of this writing he is still alive and probably taking antiretroviral drugs to prevent the onset of AIDS.

The year was 1991, and now as I look back, it was clear that even our ten-year-olds knew about the AIDS menace. In the previous decade medical experts had been gradually learning more and more about this horrific pandemic, and they were getting ready for a long battle to solve health care's gigantic problem. Our knowledge base about the disease grew slowly.

THE EARLY YEARS

First, there were reports sent to the Centers for Disease Control and Prevention (CDC) about a strange illness observed by physicians in Los Angeles and New York. In the summer of 1981 the CDC documented five cases of a rare form of pneumonia in Los Angeles. All the patients were described as previously healthy young men who happened to be homosexuals, and two of them had died. The medical literature refers to these events as the "beginning of AIDS in the U.S." Other reports about peculiar illnesses from New York and San Francisco came in with unique but similar features. A rare form of skin cancer called "Kaposi's sarcoma" occurred among gay men in New York. Within a year and a half the CDC had concluded that they were dealing with a cellular-immune dysfunction. The term "AIDS" would not be coined until 1982, but by 1990 the World Health Organization (WHO) called the situation what it was: a world pandemic. With that label, scientists were telling us that AIDS was unquestionably an epidemic that had jumped continents.[2] Everyone was expected to take appropriate action to prevent the spread of this disease. Some were more capable than others at taking meaningful action recommended by public health experts.

Those who were interested signed up for a crash course on this new and dangerous disease called Acquired Immunodeficiency Syndrome (AIDS). No one actually knew what caused the disorder until 1983 when two French virologists discovered that this infectious disease was brought about by a unique virus, which they eventually called the human immunodeficiency virus (HIV). Francoise Barré-Sinoussi and Luc Montagnier of the Pasteur Institute, Paris, France, received the Nobel Prize in 2008 for their scientific breakthrough.[3] Soon after the French discovery of the virus that causes AIDS, Dr. Robert Gallo of the National Cancer Institute developed the first test to detect HIV in April 1984 using blood samples. Thus, after three years of intense research the CDC was able to inform the medical community that there now was a test for HIV, which can lead to AIDS and death unless treated.[4] Moreover, Gallo's work gave the CDC and the Red Cross a test that could be used to screen blood for HIV contamination, so the problem of "killer blood" was resolved as well.

During the first twenty years of AIDS research, scientists found that a small percentage of people (< 5 percent) carrying the HIV virus showed little or no signs of damage despite having been infected for many years. They have been given the name long-term survivors (LTS) and their good fortune seems to be the result of superior genes and virus genotype (weak).[5] Medical surveillance teams at work throughout the country, however, found that many Americans were not so lucky. The precise number of AIDS cases identified in the United States by February 1985 according to the CDC was 8,495, and 4,077 were already dead (47.9 percent).[6] Two years later some 50,000 Americans had become infected with HIV/AIDs (see table 2.1). Panic was not the proper word to use at this time, but families, doctors and public officials were gravely concerned.

By the time the data in table 2.1 were published by CDC analysts, the majority of those diagnosed with AIDS had died. At this point, U.S. Surgeon General Dr. C. Everett Koop voiced his concerns about HIV/AIDS.

Table 2.1. The cumulative number and percentage of persons with HIV/AIDS in the United States, 1981–1987.

Gender	*N*	*Percentage*
Male	46,251	92
Female	4,029	8
Total	50,280	100

Source: CDC, *Morbidity and Mortality Weekly Report* 50, no. 21 (June 1, 2001): 431 [Historical review].

His office wanted everyone to realize that this was a very deadly disease. The message was inescapable: move fast in order to save lives. As we have observed above, medical science was doing the heavy lifting at this stage, but there were many problems left to be resolved.

With about 90 percent of U.S. AIDS cases coming from the male population during the early years, the CDC developed a model for a typical disease trajectory beginning with mostly males contracting HIV, and with no miracle drug for a cure, expectations regarding death rates were very high. With most victims getting the virus through sexual contact, intravenous drug use,[7] or blood transfusions, the disease brought death to many. For some, however, the disease remained in a latent stage for many years with no real symptoms of any kind. During this time period the HIV-positive person was capable of transmitting the virus to numerous people long before they were tested or became sick enough for the victim to see a doctor for examination, diagnosis, and treatment. Thus, two important policies were stressed by the CDC, UNAIDS, and other prevention programs: (1) people should get tested for HIV / AIDS and (2) they should use a condom when having sex. The rationale was fairly obvious: if a person knows he or she is HIV positive, he or she would hopefully avoid having sexual relations without protection. The hope among public health experts was that the normal ethical standard ingrained in most human beings would kick in and get the virus carrier to look out for the health of the person they might infect. So testing was key to prevention. Nevertheless, these two prevention items—testing and the use of condoms—were not easy to implement even in high income countries like the United States; they were even more of a problem for developing countries like Africa, where AIDS was most prevalent.

As the disease took its usual course, for the vast majority of HIV positive subjects before 1990, there was a gradual suppression of the body's immune system, which led to noticeable medical conditions that could be treated only to a moderate degree. The key is early detection. Generally, the transition from HIV to full-blown AIDS is associated with chronic fevers, night sweats, swollen glands, and unexplained weight loss, to mention just some of the signs of the disease. In the later stages of AIDS the patient may experience bouts with pneumonia, skin cancer, seizures, and finally death. With the advent and use of new and powerful antiretroviral drugs, the AIDS patient can live much longer than was previously thought possible. Gregory L. Weiss and Lynn E. Lonnquist make this clear: "While average life expectancy in the 1990s for someone with AIDS in the United States was about ten years, by mid-2000, it was more than twenty years."[8] Once again we see how science intervenes and improves the human condition. But on the downside, the cost for these antiretroviral drugs that keep people alive can be as much as $7,000–$8,000 per year.[9] Many did not have access to such medications nor could they afford to buy them. AIDS for them was a death sentence.

During the early period of research, the AIDS crisis occasioned important scientific breakthroughs that helped health care workers fight the disease. At first there were mistakes and a great deal of confusion. Due to the small number of cases the CDC had to work with initially, some researchers thought that the disease was peculiar to homosexuals only. The first manifestation of the disease occurred in gay men; thus Robert O. Brennan and David T. Durack[10] took the view in 1981 that the medical profession was dealing with some sort of gay disease. But soon such theories were rejected when children who were hemophiliacs developed AIDS due to contaminated blood transfusions. Moreover, research on newborns who acquired AIDS from their infected mothers prompted scholars to throw the "gay man" hypothesis out the window. Anyone could contract the disease if exposed to the virus; everyone was at risk, some more than others. During the early years, however, Dr. C. Everett Koop kept emphasizing that one cannot get AIDS through casual contact, but only through semen, vaginal secretions, or blood. Despite these caveats, AIDS-phobia became a part of American life. This was exemplified by the case of Ryan White, who was banned from his Indiana middle school because he had AIDS. Ryan, a hemophiliac, contracted the virus through a blood transfusion and eventually died in 1990 at age eighteen.[11] He did not live long enough to benefit from the antiretroviral drugs that were just coming on the market in 1989–1990.

NEED FOR PREVENTION

Prevention programs became a top priority during 1984–1987 as well as the need to solve the blood contamination problem; a significant number of hemophiliacs had gotten AIDS from contaminated blood donated unwittingly by diseased citizens, and many patients died. By 1985 health officials reported that they knew of 113 cases of AIDS linked to blood or blood products.[12] U.S. tennis great Arthur Ashe died of AIDS in 1993 at age fifty, but medical investigations into the cause of his death concluded that he acquired the disease from a blood transfusion while undergoing heart surgery in 1983. Lag time from infection to death: ten years. The term "killer blood" took on an ominous connotation and became a popular term among journalists at this time. By January 1985, the FDA approved the first test to screen blood and blood products for HIV. Government programs already mandated the screening of the nation's blood supply for "hepatitis B," so checking for HIV would soon become a routine task for the Red Cross and other agencies in charge of the blood supply. The idea of developing a vaccine to prevent the disease was a long way off then and still is. The CDC made it clear to the medical community that there now was a test for HIV, which can lead to AIDS and death unless treated.[13] Now medical science had a test to find out if humans had the HIV virus and determine if a given sample of blood was safe.

Prevention programs in the United States took center stage as Dr. C. Everett Koop, the surgeon general under President Reagan, stressed the need for education and knowledge of condom use to limit the spread of AIDS. By 1986–1987 it was clear to him and to the scientific community that the majority of HIV/AIDS cases occurred due to sexual contact. The most current data (2006–2009) we have on how people in the United States contract the disease are found in figure 2.1.

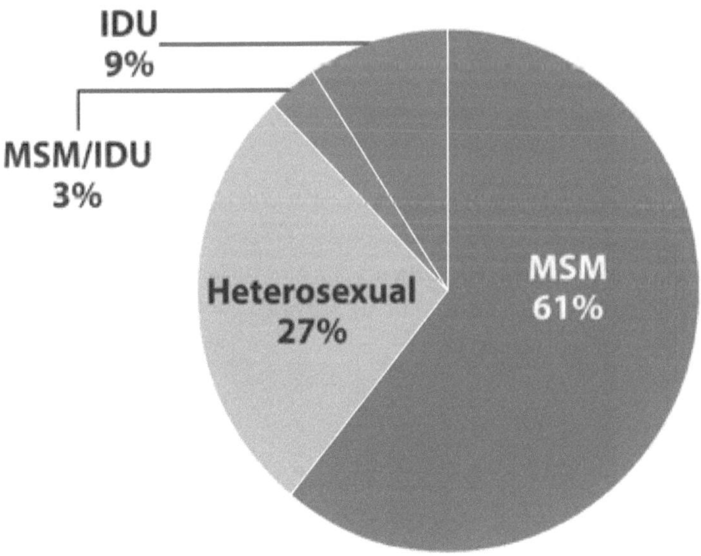

Figure 2.1. Estimated New HIV Infections, 2009, by Transmission Category. Used by permission of J. Prejean, R. Song, A. Hernandez, R. Ziebell, T. Green, et al. (2011).

Although the sources of infection have varied somewhat over the years, the main point of the CDC and Dr. Koop from the very beginning was this: the vast majority of new HIV infections were the result of sexual contact, that is, HIV infected men who have sex with men (MSM), 61 percent; heterosexual contact, 27 percent; intravenous drug users (IDU) played a relatively minor role. Currently, we know that almost 90 percent of all new cases of HIV are from some kind of sexual contact. Intravenous drug use (IDU) comprises 9 percent of the new cases according to CDC reports on the United States. At the time of Dr. Koop's tenure, the disease was spreading fast at home and abroad, and no one knew what the exact trajectory of the HIV/AIDS disease would be for the next ten years.

From hindsight one can see that Dr. Koop was on the right track in the 1980s, but not everyone supported his education program that included seminars on the importance of using condoms when having sex.

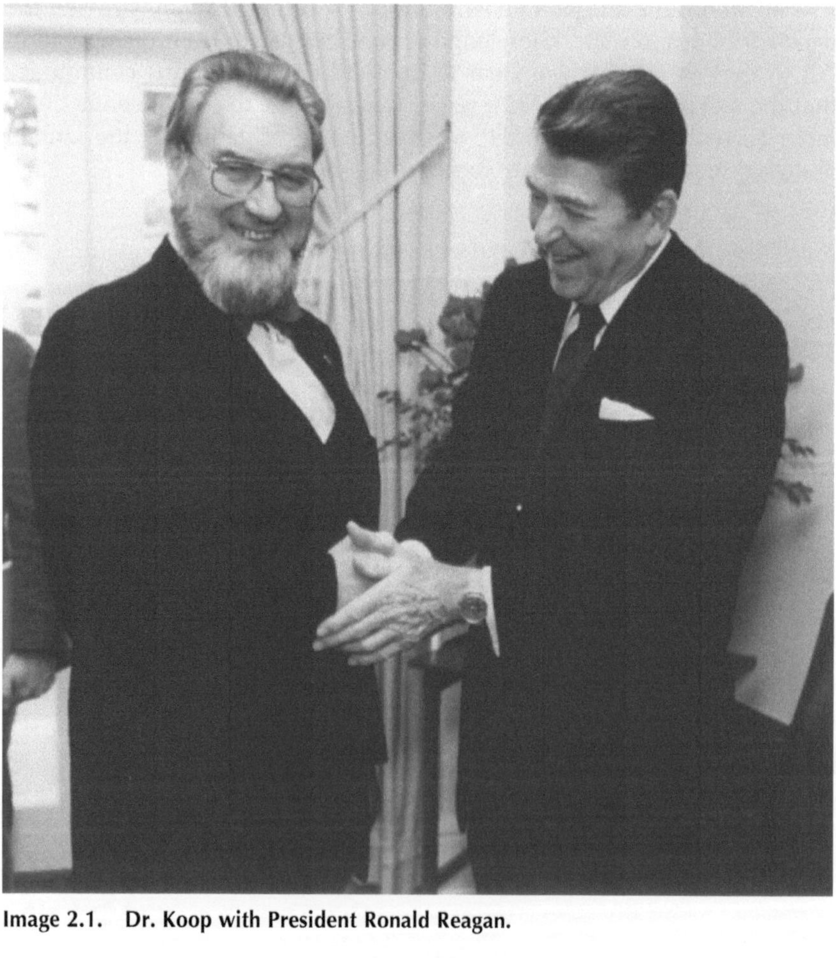

Image 2.1. Dr. Koop with President Ronald Reagan.

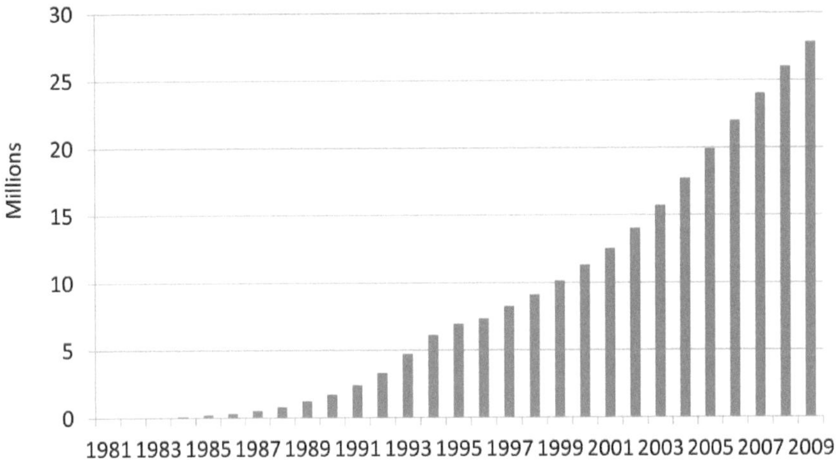

Figure 2.2. Cumulative AIDS Deaths Worldwide, 1981–2009. UNAIDS, Global Report, 2010.

His detractors called him the "Condom King," and they objected to his sex education program. In his defense we should point out that he advocated abstinence and fidelity first, but when people would not adhere to this simple prevention program, he emphasized the use of condoms.[14] He wanted to save lives, but many of his critics just did not want to talk about sex and AIDS. Perhaps he had an inkling about what was happening on the international scene, and he wanted to guard against contagion in the United States as much as possible. Whatever his inner light was telling him, Koop's public policy recommendations were truly insightful (see figure 2.2).

Few saw the explosive nature of the HIV virus like Dr. Koop, whose medical insights curbed the spread of AIDS in the United States. But managing the AIDS problem on the world stage would be a much more difficult assignment. Figure 2.2 shows that in the next twenty years (1987–2007), AIDS deaths sky rocketed. It is evident that secular leaders in the West moved quickly in the early 1980s to deal with the AIDS crisis. But the task was extremely complicated due to the intractable nature of human institutions and the people who run them. Early on deaths due to AIDS were minimal, but by the end of the 1990s, casualties were about twelve million worldwide. In the United States, however, the number of deaths due to AIDS fell from 49,895 in 1995 to 14,215 four years later (1999).[15] The U.S. trends were moving in the opposite direction of global statistics. Less than one-half of one percent (<0.5 percent) of AIDS deaths throughout the world took place in the United States, but its total population at the time constituted about 4.2 percent of those living on the planet. The disease of AIDS was under-represented in the United States, compared to other countries dealing with HIV. Something was working.

ANTIRETROVIRAL DRUGS

The early U.S. trends can be seen in figure 2.3 below. While poorer countries seemed helpless in controlling HIV/AIDS, the United States, Canada, and Europe benefited from new sets of drug treatments that slowed the progression of AIDS. Obviously there was no cure for AIDS at this time. With the introduction of the first FDA approved antiretroviral drug (AZT) in 1987, the HIV/AIDS treatment program took a major step in the direction of reducing the number of people going from testing positive for HIV to developing full-blown AIDS and dying.[16] With AZT[17] on the market by 1989 and in major usage by 1991–1992, medical experts looked for data to show that AIDS deaths were declining due to the introduction of this new drug. They would not be disappointed. Clinical trials showed that AZT safely prolongs the lives of patients who test positive for HIV.[18] CDC data revealed that AZT was truly a success story: yearly AIDS incidence declined significantly. The major problem was its price tag: a year's supply of AZT in 1990 could cost a patient $7,000, and not all insurance companies would pay for this new, innovative treatment.

Despite the fact that AZT was at first available to only a limited number of patients in the United States, one can observe its power to limit the progression of AIDS in the HIV positive group (figure 2.3). Certainly, other factors were at work as well. By 1995 a second antiretroviral drug was approved by the FDA, and this new treatment program (protease inhibitors) proved to be even more important in the fight against AIDS. It slowed the development to full-blown AIDS, and there were fewer negative side effects—always a problem with AZT. These new drugs considerably reduced the pain and suffering for AIDS patients. Today, those

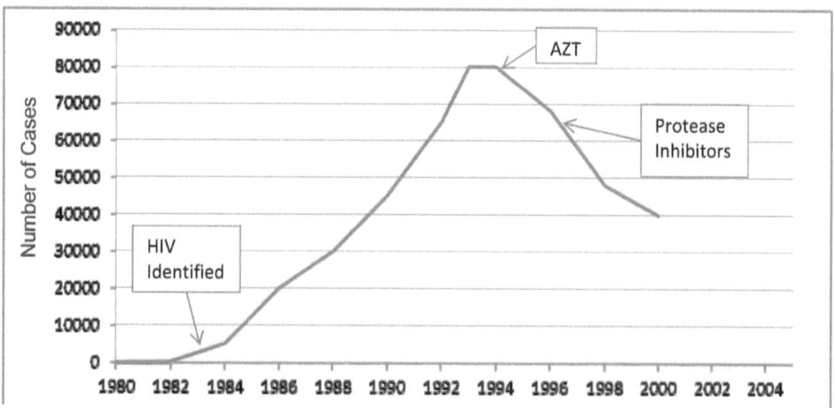

Figure 2.3. Estimated AIDS Incidence through 2000, United States. Estimated from data reported to CDC through June 2001.

with HIV / AIDS can benefit from over twenty new antiretroviral drugs, but unfortunately large numbers of patients in developing countries do not have access to such treatments. Clinical studies have shown that a combination of several antiretroviral drugs, called "highly active antiretroviral therapy" (HAART) is the most effective approach in treating HIV / AIDS.[19] In contrast to the U.S. experience, we find in sub-Saharan Africa that only about 49 percent of those in need of antiretroviral drugs actually receive the treatment.[20] This number would be much lower if it were not for the PEPFAR program initiated by George W. Bush in 2003. The President's Emergency Plan for AIDS Relief (PEPFAR) allocated $18.8 billion for years 2003–2008 to help fifteen countries deal with the HIV / AIDS crisis. The program design included twelve countries in Africa, one of which was South Africa. Bishop Kevin Dowling of Rustenburg, South Africa, told me in a private interview that he was grateful for this medical aid and reports it has saved many lives in his diocese. About half of the PEPFAR funds are used to pay for antiretroviral drugs which help sick people keep their jobs, serve their families, and extend life.[21] Evaluation studies show that in the twelve African PEPFAR countries there has been a 10.5 percent reduction in death rates due to AIDS, compared to neighboring countries without PEPFAR. In concrete terms, that means 1.2 million deaths have been averted because of PEPFAR's activities funded by the United States. Before he left office, Bush was able to convince Congress to extend funding for this AIDS intervention project until 2013 with an additional $48 billion.[22] Antiretroviral drugs were introduced to the United States, Canada, and Europe in the early 1990s, but it took about ten years for these miracle drugs to reach hard-hit developing nations. We have heard about trickle-down economics; this is trickle-down health care. Many in the poorer countries of the world died before modern medicine arrived on the scene. Before 2003, doctors in sub-Saharan Africa observed that HIV's usual course is to disable the immune system. This process allows normally controllable infections to overcome the body's defenses and kill the person. The new drugs changed that scenario to some degree.

CONCLUSION

This overview shows that Dr. C. Everett Koop was a pioneer in developing programs to deal with AIDS in the United States during the 1980s. Later on President George W. Bush helped fight AIDS on the international scene with PEPFAR. Koop's years of experience as a practicing physician paid off in the early stages of program development during the AIDS crisis. Bush, with his faith-based public policy initiative, reached out to those in dire need and helped many who were suffering the most. Koop's quick thinking and planning helped to limit AIDS infections and deaths in the United States while poorer countries languished with little hope of controlling the disease until about 2003. For example, approximately thirty-four million people were living with HIV/AIDS worldwide in 2010 with 67 percent of these victims residing in sub-Saharan Africa. The United States and other developed countries have been able to slow down the AIDS crisis at home. Much more work still needs to be done abroad.

Obviously, things were getting out of control on the international scene by the mid-1990s. The U.S. experience demonstrated that prevention programs based on lifestyle changes (abstinence, fidelity) and the use of condoms saved lives. The Koop program was controversial, but many states and local communities took up the challenge despite pockets of opposition. Health education programs in major cities provided free condoms and clean needles for drug users. Many citizens did not like that approach, but in the end anything that would save lives and control a deadly disease trumped the conservative backlash. It was a whole new ball game and the rules had to change somewhat.

There were about thirty-four million persons in the world living with HIV/AIDS in 2010, with approximately 2.7 million new cases emerging each year. Only 6.6 million people were receiving antiretroviral therapy in low- and middle-income countries.[23] Hence, there was a tremendous need for drug intervention in developing countries. The UNAIDS 2011 reports reveal that approximately 30 [range 25 to 33] million people have died from AIDS since health experts began tracking the disease around 1981. The United States had about 1.2 million people living with HIV/AIDS in 2009, and roughly 310,000 of them were women.[24] Despite the many years of substantial progress in treating AIDS, the number of new HIV infections has remained relatively constant: around 50,000 per year in the United States since the mid-1990s; an estimated 47,500 people became newly infected with the virus in 2010. The CDC estimates that about 20 percent of those afflicted with HIV/AIDS in the United States are unaware that they are carrying the disease.[25] Mortality statistics reveal that from 1981 through 2007, about 570,000 persons in the United States have perished from AIDS. The work to deal with this problem has only just begun.

NOTES

1. Many writers use the more technically correct term "test positive for HIV," but I prefer the commonly accepted terminology "test positive for the HIV virus."

2. According to the CDC an epidemic occurs when more cases of a disease arise than is normally expected within a specific place or group of people over a given period of time. By 1985 AIDS was defined as an epidemic in the United States.

3. Lawrence Altman, "Discoverers of AIDS and Cancer Viruses Win Nobel," *New York Times*, October 7, 2008.

4. Lawrence Altman, "Blood Supply Called Free of Aids," *New York Times*, August 1, 1985, 1A.

5. David Rhodes et al., "Characterization of Three Nef-Defective Immunodeficiency Virus Type 1 Strains," *Journal of Virology* 74, no. 22 (2000): 10581–88.

6. "Hemophiliacs Immune Abnormalities," AP News Archive, February 22, 1985; also see Robert Pear, "AIDS Blood Test to Be Available in 2 to 6 Weeks," *New York Times*, March 3, 1985, 1A.

7. Some prefer the phrase "injecting drug use," and it is perhaps the better term.

8. Gregory L. Weiss and Lynne E. Lonnquist, *The Sociology of Health, Healing, and Illness*, 7th ed. (New York: Prentice Hall, 2012), 85.

9. Donald McNeil, "AIDS: A Price Break for Antiretroviral Drugs in 70 of the World's Poorest Countries," *New York Times*, May 23, 2011.

10. Robert O. Brennan and David T. Durack, "Gay Compromise Syndrome," *The Lancet* 318, no. 8259 (1981): 1338–39.

11. Dirk Johnson, "Ryan White Dies of AIDS at 18; His Struggle Helped Pierce Myths," *New York Times*, April 9, 1990.

12. Pear, "AIDS Blood Test," 1A.

13. Altman, "Blood Supply," 1A.

14. Dr. Koop's philosophy and program is laid out here: http://iml.dartmouth.edu/koop/aids/index.html (accessed May 18, 2012).

15. William Cockerham, *Medical Sociology*, 12th ed. (New York: Prentice Hall, 2012), 39.

16. Since HIV is classified as a retrovirus, scientists needed a unique drug to counteract the AIDS virus. The new antiretroviral drugs suppress the HIV infection but do not cure the victim of the disease.

17. AZT's full name is "azidothymidine" and was the first antiretroviral drug used to treat HIV/AIDS. It slows the replication of the virus in patients.

18. M. A. Fischl et al., "The Efficacy of Azidothymidine (AZT) in the Treatment of Patients with AIDS and AIDS-Related Complex. A Double-Blind, Placebo-Controlled Trial," *New England Journal of Medicine* 317, no. 4 (1987): 185–91.

19. See discussion on HAART: www.nlm.nih.gov/medlineplus/ency/article/000594.htm (accessed May 22, 2012).

20. UNAIDS, "Global HIV/AIDS Response—Progress Report 2011"; www.unaids.org/en/resources/publications/2011/name,64437,en.asp (accessed June 9, 2013).

21. Eran Bendavid and Jayanta Bhattacharya, "The President's Emergency Plan for AIDS Relief in Africa: an Evaluation of Outcomes," *Annals of Internal Medicine* 150, no. 10 (2009): 688–95.

22. "PEPFAR's Success," *Washington Post*, April 9, 2009.

23. UNAIDS, "Global HIV/AIDS," 2011.

24. University of California, San Francisco, HIV knowledge base; http://hivinsite.ucsf.edu/global?page=cr07-us-00 (accessed June 9, 2012).

25. CDC, "HIV and the United States at a Glance"; www.cdc.gov/hiv/resources/factsheets/us.htm (accessed November 4, 2012); also see "Estimates of new HIV infections in the United States, 2007–2010" (CDC, 2012).

3

Catholics and AIDS

Secular leaders throughout the world had made considerable progress in dealing with the AIDS crisis. Scientists discovered the virus that causes AIDS. Dr. Koop developed a policy to fight the disease and secured funding for research to find a cure. George W. Bush became an advocate for third world AIDS intervention programs. As Americans and the Centers for Disease Control geared up for the continued onslaught against AIDS, Catholics spent much of 1987 preparing for a special visitor: Pope John Paul II. On September 10, 1987, his Air Italia jetliner touched down at Miami International Airport to begin a ten-day pilgrimage to various cities throughout the United States. President Ronald Reagan and his wife Nancy were standing by to greet the leader of the Roman Catholic Church who was about to complete his tenth year as pope. It is well-known that his visits to countries around the world cost millions, but many believe the overall goodwill and spiritual lift the pope brought to his followers was worth the cost. Nonetheless, it should not go unnoticed that for every day the pope spends in the United States it could cost the local church about $1 million.[1] There must have been a sense of shared solidarity between these two men as their eyes met; both had suffered gunshot wounds some years previously and lived to tell about it. They were wounded but not bowed.

Journalists like to remind us that Pope John Paul II was the most traveled pontiff of all time, having visited 117 countries (some more than once) during his long reign—1978 to 2005. However, not all had gone according to script for the second papal visit to the United States. On the eve of John Paul's visit, the Vatican's social communication director, Archbishop John

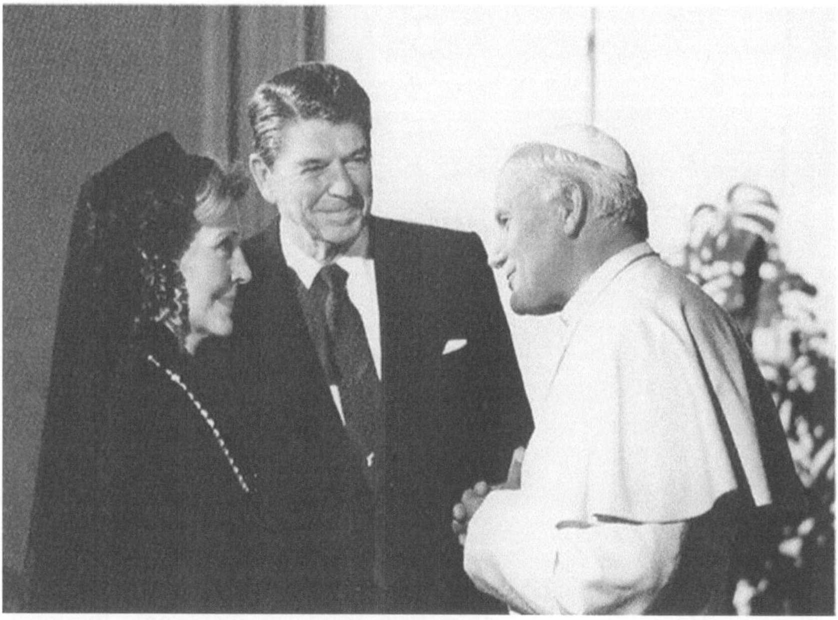

Image 3.1. Nancy and Ronald Reagan, John Paul II.

Foley, declared, "The deadly AIDS disease is a form of natural selection against homosexuals."[2] The gay community was incensed by his remarks because they took the comment to mean that God was punishing them for violating the natural law. The year before the pope's visit, Cardinal Joseph Ratzinger likewise offended many homosexuals with this observation: "Even when the practice of homosexuality may seriously threaten the lives and well-being of a large number of people, its advocates remain undeterred and refuse to consider the magnitude of the risks involved."[3] Commentators took this as a veiled reference to AIDS. Scientists had made the mistake of labeling AIDS a gay disease five years previously but had moved away from that theory rather quickly. For some reason church clerics did not get the memo. Foley's 2011 obituary in the *New York Times* did not omit the fact that he "once referred to AIDS as God's sanction against homosexual activities."[4] Later on during his visit, John Paul tried to distance himself from Foley's insensitive remarks by saying the church was doing all that was possible to heal and prevent this disease.

In San Francisco John Paul met with AIDS patients and workers at the Mission Dolores Basilica, and said: "God loves you! God loves you all, without distinction, without limit. He loves those of you who are elderly, who feel the burden of the years. He loves those of you who are sick, those who are suffering from AIDS and from AIDS-Related Complex. He loves the relatives and friends of the sick and those who care for them.

He loves us all with an unconditional and everlasting love."[5] The tone of the pope in his speeches had always been warm, friendly, and compassionate. His public policy statements, however, lacked realistic solutions to world-class problems.

Since 1981 Pope John Paul had been relatively quiet about the spread of AIDS throughout the world and offered few insights for Catholics on how to respond to this epidemic. His standard statement on how to fight AIDS was through abstinence and fidelity; he rejected the notion that Catholics could use condoms to prevent the spread of AIDS. So the entire Koop program for the United States would not be supported by Catholic Church officials.

Later that year, after the pope had returned to Rome, the U.S. Conference of Catholic Bishops would speak out on AIDS prevention and treatment. On November 14, 1987, the administrative board of the U.S. Catholic Bishops published a document called "The Many Faces of AIDS: A Gospel Response," which demonstrated pastoral concern for the problem and suggested that information about condoms[6] might be included in education programs aimed at preventing AIDS. They wrote,

> We recognize that public educational programs addressed to a wide audience will reflect the fact that some people will not act as they can and should; that they will not refrain from the type of sexual or drug-abuse behavior that can transmit AIDS. In such situations, educational efforts, if grounded in the broader moral vision outlined above, could include accurate information about prophylactic devices or other practices proposed by some medical experts as potential means of preventing AIDS.[7]

Some would see in this communique a vague reference to Dr. Koop's initiative to prevent AIDS (see table 3.1). The surgeon general's office was in Washington, D.C., and so was the U.S. Catholic Bishops' central headquarters. It looked as though these two groups had shared ideas to some degree. Statements by the U.S. bishops give pastors and Catholic leaders insights about what they should do in a crisis situation. AIDS was a social issue that needed to be addressed. Nevertheless, Cardinal Joseph Ratzinger (elected Pope Benedict XVI in 2005), prefect of the powerful Congregation for the Doctrine of the Faith, wrote a letter to the American bishops in 1988 which appeared to chide them "for having issued their

Table 3.1. Catholic Church policy and the Koop program compared.

	Koop	*Catholic Church*
Abstinence	Yes	Yes
Fidelity	Yes	Yes
Use Condoms	Yes	No

earlier statement without consulting Rome and warned against the appearance of condoning immoral practices."[8] The U.S. bishops were the first to challenge Rome on its refusal to allow Catholics to use condoms to prevent AIDS. But in the minds of Cardinal Ratzinger and the pope, there were some things that Catholics just could not do.

Two years later the Catholic Church held its first conference in Rome devoted to the AIDS crisis. The November 1989 meeting featured conservative speakers like Cardinal John O'Conner of New York, and many were wondering what he would say, given the 1987 bishops' pastoral statement regarding AIDS. He did not disappoint Vatican hardliners. O'Conner quickly condemned the use of condoms to prevent the spread of AIDS and similarly rejected the idea of distributing clean syringes to drug addicts. It was no surprise to critical thinking American Catholics, therefore, when the full body of U.S. bishops issued a new AIDS statement and dropped its earlier "conditional support for condom education in schools and urged that AIDS prevention emphasize chastity instead."[9] By 1989 battle lines were drawn and the new bishops' letter, "Called to Compassion and Responsibility," was an example of socio-religious reentrenchment. The Roman Catholic Church's centralized administration asserted that the way to fight AIDS would be through abstinence and fidelity, not condoms. The American Bishops' Conference had been pressured to conform to Rome's policy that many found difficult to justify.

With Pope John Paul II in charismatic control and Cardinal Ratzinger pillorying theological dissidents since his appointment in 1981, the church's general policy regarding the non-use of condoms to fight the spread of AIDS had remained relatively unchallenged by cardinals and bishops. Some U.S. bishops tried to offer a new direction in 1987 under the leadership of Cardinal Joseph Bernardin, but that initiative was thwarted. In the words of sociological theorists Fligstein and McAdam the *incumbents* in the Catholic organization had taken control of the church and defined what was acceptable teaching and behavior. These sociologists view incumbents as actors within an organization who "wield disproportionate influence" and try to maintain the status quo whenever possible.[10] This certainly is what happened to Catholic Church policy in the 1980s. Nonetheless, there were others in the Catholic organization who tried to gain power and influence in order to bring about change. The *challengers* emerge from time to time and question the teaching, directives, and policy of incumbents and this brings about some organizational conflict. Challengers "occupy less privileged niches within the field and ordinarily wield little influence over its operation."[11] They usually articulate an alternative vision of the organization. For the next twenty years the Catholic Church would debate at the highest levels of the Vatican whether condoms could be used to prevent the spread of AIDS. The U.S. Catholic bishops challenged Rome's stand and were rebuffed. Church policy in the 1980s adhered to the simple formula: A + B and no C. That is, abstain from sex, be faithful, but above all, no condoms. As AIDS became more and more of a global health problem, other actors would emerge on the scene to oppose papal pronouncements. The U.S. challengers could have easily recalled the words of the great father of the American Revolution, John Paul Jones: "I have not yet begun to fight." The war of words would inspire others.

NOTES

1. Neela Banerjee, "Hefty Bill for Pope's Visit Looms for Archdioceses," *New York Times*, April 14, 2008.
2. *Milwaukee Sentinel*, September 10, 1987. Also see Robert Reinhold, "The Papal Visit; AIDS Issue at Fore as Pope Visits San Francisco Today," *New York Times*, September 17, 1987.
3. Cardinal Joseph Ratzinger, "Letter to the Bishops of the Catholic Church on the Pastoral Care of Homosexual Persons," Congregation for the Doctrine of the Faith, Rome, October 1, 1986.
4. Douglas Martin, "Cardinal John P. Foley, 76, Vatican Spokesman, Dies," *New York Times*, December 12, 2011.
5. John Paul II, Address at Mission Dolores Basilica, San Francisco, California, September 17, 1987.
6. The statement used the term prophylactics, a generic term which includes a host of contraceptive devices, including condoms.
7. U.S. Catholic Bishops Administrative Board, "The Many Faces of AIDS: A Gospel Response," Washington, D.C., November 14, 1987.
8. Quoted in Peter Steinfels, "Catholic Bishops Vote to Retain Controversial Statement on AIDS," *New York Times*, June 28, 1988.
9. "Vatican AIDS Meeting Hears O'Connor Assail Condom Use," *New York Times*, November 14, 1989.
10. Neil Fligstein and Doug McAdam, "Toward a General Theory of Strategic Action Fields," *Sociological Theory* 29, no. 1 (2011): 5.
11. Fligstein and McAdam, "Toward a General Theory," 6.

4

The Continent and AIDS

Europe Did Not Sleep

By the mid-1980s Western Europe was beginning to feel the impact of the AIDS pandemic. Between 1985 and 1991, this region reported a major increase in newly diagnosed HIV cases, that is, a twenty-one fold change from 5,000 to 112,000 victims in six years.[1] Central and Eastern Europe were mostly free from HIV during this period. We will see later that the Catholic Church there did not stand by in silence in the face of this crisis.[2] But by 2005 the total number of those living with HIV/AIDS had jumped to 820,000—considerably less than comparable numbers in the United States: 1,200,000.[3] With the introduction of antiretroviral drugs in the region, the death rates were relatively low (figure 4.1).

Europe and the United States together had about two million victims of HIV/AIDS (about 7 percent of the worldwide total), but they represented about 95 percent of the research and scientific discoveries on how to deal with the new disease. Between 1981 and 1990, Europe felt the initial brunt of this modern plague. The introduction of antiretroviral drugs to deal with HIV/AIDS helped to keep death rates down in the 1990s, but all signs indicated things were going to get worse before they got better. Something had to be done and done quickly. By 2010 the numbers skyrocketed to close to a million in the region. The trajectory of the disease was clear after almost three decades.

Without question, Europe was not being hit by AIDS like the United States as is evident in table 4.1. But over the years, victims of the disease added up and some countries were hit harder than others.

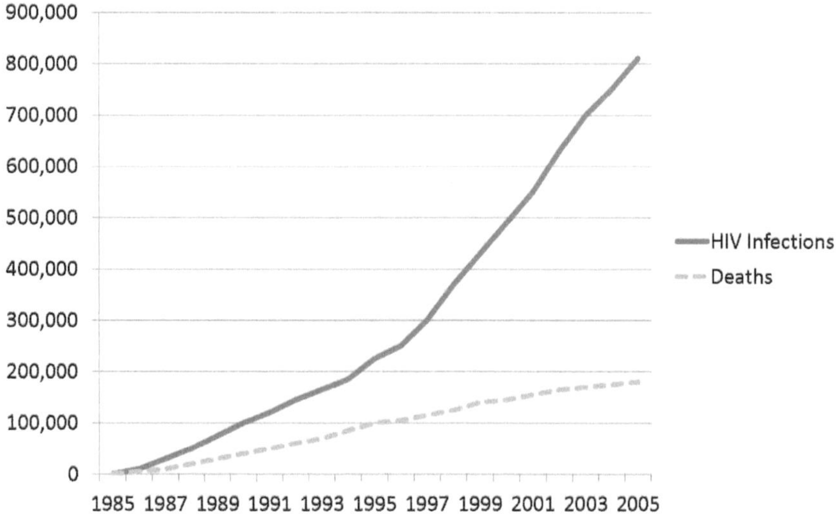

Figure 4.1. HIV/AIDS Data for Europe, 1985–2005. UNAIDS, Global Report, 2010.

Switzerland and France were hit hardest, but nothing like the spread of AIDS in other parts of the world.[4] Prior to 1990, Catholic Church officials in France had begun to take notice of the ever-increasing rise in HIV/AIDS cases, and so Cardinal Jean-Marie Lustiger, Archbishop of Paris, spoke out regarding the world epidemic. In 1988 he advocated the use of condoms for those who had tested positive for the AIDS virus.[5] We do not know if he had been reading some of the press clippings from the United States, or the 1987 bishops' statement, "The Many Faces of AIDS," but his message resonated with the American bishops' stance. The church in France had to speak out. Lustiger was the first high-ranking European cleric to offer an alternative to the Vatican two-step plan of abstinence and fidelity. Soon after, another French bishop, Jacques

Table 4.1. Cumulative AIDS incidence rates per million population, Europe, 1990.

Country	*Rate*
Switzerland	190.2
France	173.2
Spain	135.1
Denmark	112.4
Italy	105.3
United States	**515.7**

Source: CDC, *Morbidity and Mortality Weekly Report*, November 30, 1990.

Gaillot, followed suit by telling Catholics that he approved the use of contraceptives as a precaution against AIDS.[6] The increasing number of AIDS cases in France by the end of the 1980s probably motivated these local bishops to consider an alternative to the Vatican policy. Although the problem was not as serious as the U.S. outbreak when controlling for population differences (see table 4.1), church officials in France felt that it was their obligation to alert Catholics to the regional and global complexities of HIV/AIDS. Soon after the French challenge, Vatican officials probably began work on an encyclical to deal with this situation. Pope John Paul II apparently did not like the way some of his fellow bishops were reacting to the AIDS crisis. The bishop of Rome decided he had to respond to the bishops in the Diaspora.

In 1993 the pope promulgated his tenth encyclical letter to Catholics; it was called *Veritatis Splendor*. Here the pope devoted a significant portion of his comments to issues related to contemporary moral theology and pointed out that certain behaviors were "intrinsically evil" and contraceptive acts were one of them.[7] Condoms were banned by church teaching, and therefore, could never be a part of the Catholic plan to fight AIDS. Case closed. It is hard to believe that the pope and his advisors were not aware of a growing church movement to try and change Catholic teaching about the use of condoms for treating infectious diseases. Consequently, John Paul II felt that it was necessary to make a strong, public statement that there would be no change even in the face of mounting AIDS casualties. The only question was, would the official Vatican statement stop the challengers? The answer is yes and no.

The reactions to this encyclical were predictable. A few voices had risen up in the church's hierarchy and stated that condoms could be used to prevent the spread of AIDS. After the 1993 promulgation of *Veritatis Splendor* there was a relatively long period of silence among the world's Catholic bishops. One of the few exceptions was Archbishop Christoph Schönborn of Austria (one of the *papabile* in 2013); he maintained that the use of condoms to fight AIDS was morally acceptable.[8] But the Vatican was not going to budge on this point.

Despite the incident in Austria, very few bishops were going to ask for a change in church teaching immediately after the pope, in effect, said "NO" to the use of condoms to prevent AIDS through a formal encyclical. Cardinal Ratzinger, known in some ecclesiastical circles at the time as the great "Enforcer," and "God's Rottweiler" would monitor the airwaves and make sure dioceses throughout the world conformed to the teaching of *Veritatis Splendor*. During this time period Vatican officials always reminded Catholics that using condoms was against papal teaching and immoral; they never raised the question of condom effectiveness. That argument would come later.

From an organizational perspective the pope's encyclical created a *dead zone* for reformers, and not many were going to raise their voices in protest—at least for a while. After all, this was not UC Berkeley in the 1960s where there were almost weekly protests against *Humanae Vitae,* and every other authoritarian pronouncement that came along. A different set of clerics and church administrators had taken over the post–Vatican II church. You could lose your job for speaking out against the pope and his policies. Liberal priests like Hans Küng and Charles Curran were relieved of their teaching duties when they opposed church teachings. There was a new sheriff in Vatican City and no one was in the mood for open conflict—at least not just yet. All was quiet on the western front for now. But one thing did change: more and more people became infected with HIV and died of AIDS. And because high-level church leaders felt bound by the teachings of previous popes, they seemed paralyzed to join forces with the international community in the fight against AIDS even when the World Health Organization (WHO), UNAIDS, and the CDC advocated the use of condoms to save lives.

With the official church focused on treatment programs for AIDS rather than effective prevention strategies, secular authorities moved forward with their own set of priorities.

1. Europeans, like their American counterparts, wanted to tackle the problem of mother-child transmission of HIV. With the help of public and private funding, the medical community set up programs to offer free HIV testing for all pregnant women. The goal was education and treatment for all those testing positive for HIV. Physician-scientists had discovered that if an expectant mother was given anti-retroviral drugs, for example, Nevirapine, during the twenty-eighth week of pregnancy, the chance that the baby would become infected with HIV was cut in half.[9] This health care initiative has been proven effective in Europe, the United States, and Africa. Mothers who tested positive for HIV were encouraged to avoid breast feeding.
2. Other prevention programs focused on needle exchange interventions for injection drug users (IDU). The Catholic Church in 1989 gave a thumbs-down to this program despite the fact that a Yale study showed that needle exchange programs reduce new HIV infections by 33 percent.[10]
3. Health care experts continued to emphasize the use of condoms to prevent the spread of HIV/AIDS.

In conclusion, with Western Europe and the United States exchanging ideas and data on how to deal with AIDS, the death toll began to decline in these areas, and HIV infections leveled off for the most part in these countries. The next step was to focus on global concerns, especially the AIDS challenge in sub-Saharan Africa.

NOTES

1. Srdan Matic et al., *HIV/AIDS in Europe* (Geneva: World Health Organization, 2006), 94.

2. Western Europe as defined here by officials at WHO: France, Germany, Austria, Ireland, Italy, Spain, Portugal, United Kingdom, Netherlands, Belgium, Sweden, Switzerland, Norway, Demark, Luxembourg, Finland, Greece, and Iceland; Central Europe: Poland, Albania, Turkey, Czech Republic, Hungary, and several others.

3. See the University of California San Francisco Medical Center, http://hivinsite.ucsf.edu/global?page=cr10-00-00 (accessed February 3, 2013).

4. CDC, 1990 Report on Europe; www.cdc.gov/mmwr/preview/mmwrhtml/00001845.htm (accessed May 24, 2012).

5. "Religion Briefs," *Los Angeles Times*, December 10, 1988.

6. See William Smith, "The Church," in *Aspects of Contemporary France*, Sheila Perry, editor (Paris: Action Press, 1989), 153.

7. John Paul II, *Veritatis Splendor* (Vatican Press, 1993): par. 80.

8. "Top Archbishop Permits Condom Use against AIDS," *The Irish Catholic*, April 11, 1996.

9. S. Lockman et al., "Response to Antiretroviral Therapy after a Single, Peripartum Dose of Nevirapine," *New England Journal of Medicine* 356 (2007): 135. Also see Donald McNeil, "AIDS Drugs to Protect Fetus," *New York Times*, January 11, 2007.

10. U.S. Government Accountability Office, "Needle Exchange Programs," March 23, 1993.

5

+

A Voice from Africa

During the late 1990s the spread of AIDS was relentless. After Pope John Paul's encyclical was published in 1993, the number of people living with HIV/AIDS nearly doubled in sub-Saharan Africa by the year 2000 (see figure 5.1). Catholics had been warned by church officials not to use condoms to prevent the spread of AIDS.

Catholic newspapers have often mentioned that the future of the church is in Latin America and Africa. The numbers support this claim to

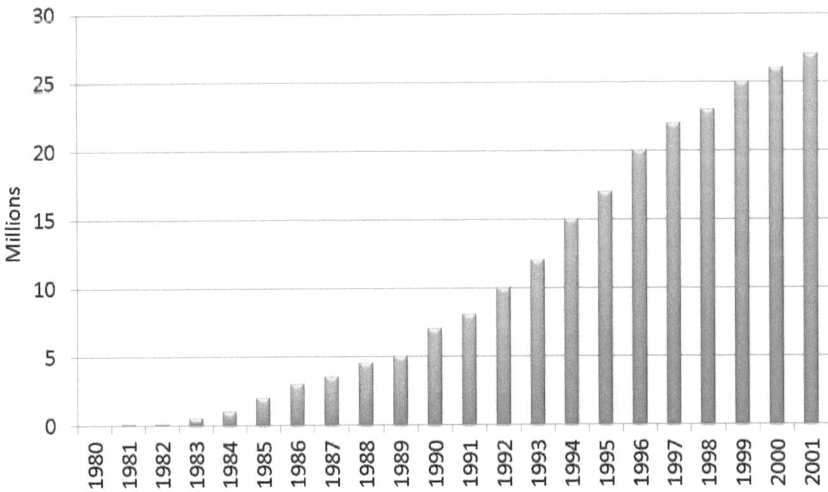

Figure 5.1. Number of People Living with HIV/AIDS in Sub-Saharan Africa, 1980–2001. UNAIDS, 2002.

some degree. The year 1978 marked the election of Cardinal Karol Wojtyla to the papacy, and with the new name "John Paul II," he heralded the growth of the African church: it was 55 million strong. The latest Vatican statistics show that there are now 150 million Catholics in Africa and this church has 33,000 priests to serve the pastoral needs of its people.[1] After Cardinal Jorge Bergoglio of Argentina was elected Pope Francis in March, 2013, it became clear that the 500 million Latin Catholics in the world were going to be heard. Africa and Latin America are centers of the Catholic Church in some respects, with 54 percent of the 1.2 billion Roman Catholics worldwide; Vatican leaders had to face this reality as AIDS ravaged its people. What would the church do for its people who were suffering in the heartland of Catholicism?

Many of those working in Catholic institutions felt helpless to do anything on the prevention side of health care. The formula to fight the disease in the United States (Dr. Koop et al.) and Europe (WHO) was simple: A + B + C. That is, to reduce the risk of getting AIDS one should practice **A**bstinence, **B**e Faithful, and use **C**ondoms. Would this program work in Africa and other developing countries? The evidence is inconclusive. There are numerous obstacles physicians and missionaries must overcome if they are to reduce the spread of HIV/AIDS in developing countries. Helen Epstein's book, *The Invisible Cure*, demonstrates that the African practice of having concurrent partners may be at the root of the problem.[2] Concurrency means simultaneous long-term sexual relationships in which friendship and trust may thwart routine condom use. The result can lead to rapid HIV infection in the group. One approach to counter this social practice is to push for abstinence and partner reduction; that is a fine idea but it is difficult to implement. When behavioral change is a low priority for couples, however, doctors and health care workers remind patients to use a condom—friend or one-night stand alike.

Catholic leaders had a problem with the third part of the ABC formula and so church members and organizations were limited on the prevention side of AIDS health care. Nevertheless, numerous health care experts, like Dr. Marcella Alsan, rightly acknowledged that Catholic "organizations mercifully provide around 25 percent of the care AIDS victims receive worldwide."[3] Since Catholics represent only about 16.9 percent of the world's population, that is a remarkable amount of service for a single religious denomination. Catholic organizations like *Caritas* perform extensive health care service around the world, specifically providing services to fourteen thousand AIDS orphans in Namibia.[4] It became evident, however, that those working in AIDS-ravaged Africa wanted to do more. Nowhere in Africa was there more of a need for AIDS prevention programs than in the diocese of Rustenburg, South Africa. It was in this small enclave, about eighty miles west of Johannesburg, that Bishop Kevin

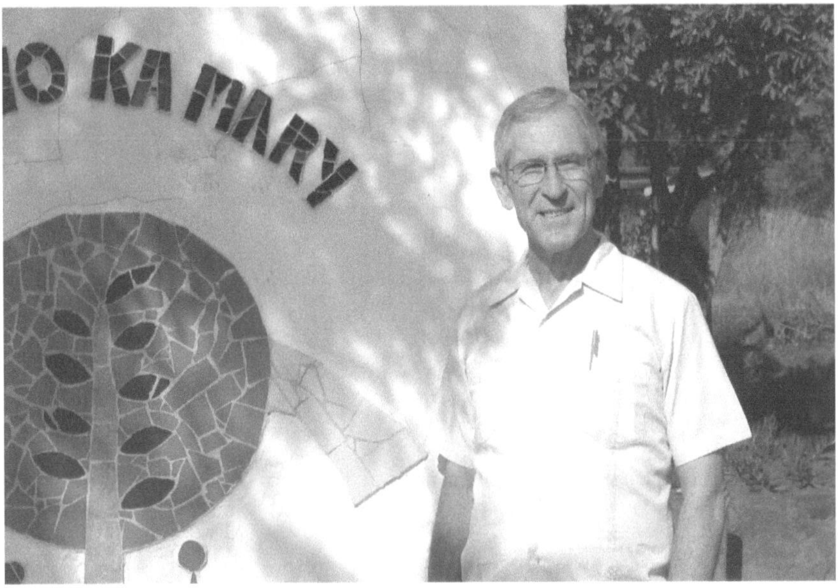

Image 5.1. Bishop Kevin Dowling visiting clinic in South Africa. Used by permission of Tara Osborne.

Dowling set up AIDS clinics to help those who were suffering and dying from the disease. The clinics served the local community—Catholics and non-Catholics alike. The day-to-day experience of AIDS led the bishop to think about the prevention side of health care but his hands were tied

AIDS was a growing problem because, among other things, the regional employment structure required large numbers of men to live away from home many months during the year to earn money to support their families in Rustenburg. Jobs in the platinum mining industry were one of the few sources of income in this region. But without hearth and home the men invariably sought out sex partners for a few moments of fleeting pleasure after a long day's work. Often the men contracted HIV/AIDS many miles away from their families, and when they had time off, they would return home for a few days. In the normal interaction of married life, wives would get AIDS from their infected husbands, suffer and then die like many others in the community. Soon both parents passed away from AIDS, and the children became orphans. Catholic Relief Services estimates that there will be about twenty million orphans due to AIDS in Africa by 2020.[5]

It is not surprising to read that AIDS is the major social problem in the world of African Christians as well as other religious groups. In sub-Saharan Africa four features of the medical landscape jump out at the world community for reflection (figure 5.2).

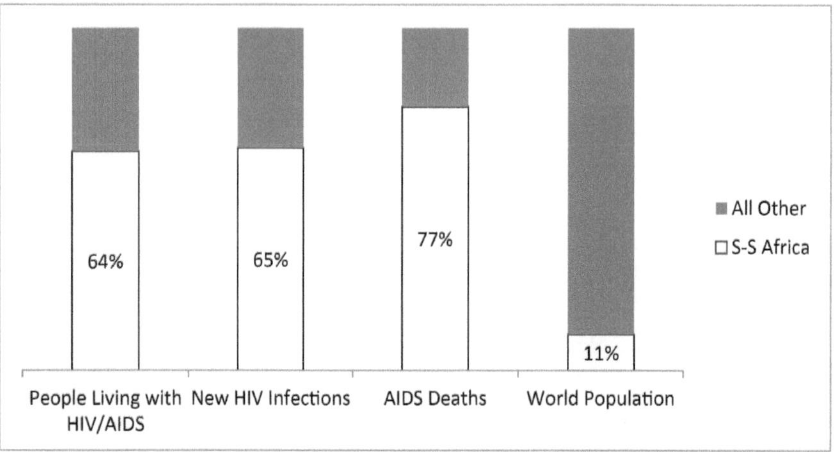

Figure 5.2. Sub-Saharan Africa as a Percentage of the Global HIV/AIDS Epidemic, 2005. The Henry J. Kaiser Family Foundation, HIV/AIDS Policy Fact Sheet, February 2006.

First, demographers point out that this region comprises only about 11 percent of the world's total population, but we find that 64 percent of all those living with HIV/AIDS worldwide reside in sub-Saharan Africa. Medical scholars like Dr. Peter Piot note that the disease probably started in Africa before 1980 and went unchecked for many years before victims in developed countries like the United States were observed, analyzed, and treated.[6] With that kind of head start the disease spread through Africa like wildfire before rich nations felt the pain of AIDS and began working on a cure. The poor have to wait for their health care. Second, funerals are a constant news story in Africa; 77 percent of all AIDS deaths in the world take place in sub-Saharan Africa. The logical step in this chaotic situation is to think prevention. How can one convince couples to use a condom when their partner has tested positive for HIV/AIDS? And yes, Catholic women should be able to use condoms to minimize their chances of contracting AIDS—that was Bishop Dowling's perspective. We heard this message from the bishops of France, the United States, and Austria before 1996.

UNAIDS data show that 60 percent of those with AIDS in sub-Saharan Africa are women—a trend markedly different from the American experience. Papal critics saw how reasonable the ABC approach would be, but how does one get the pope and the clergy in Rome to sign on? Dowling decided to go public and appealed to church officials in 2001 to respond to this emergency situation. His message was simple and to the point. The church should allow couples to use a condom to prevent the transmission of potential death to another living human being. "The use of a condom can be seen," he argued, "not as a means to prevent the 'transmission of life' leading to pregnancy, but rather as a means to prevent the 'transmission of death' to another."[7] Eight years after the encyclical *Veritatis Splendor*, Dowling took a chance that someone at the Vatican was listening. However, history was not on his side. But, he thought, perhaps the progressives in the United States and France did not use the correct approach. He was a pastor living in a territory where people were dying of AIDS every day. Certainly his words would carry more weight and the pope would listen. Not really.

Dowling was one of the first bishops in the new millennium to challenge the Vatican's stand on condoms and AIDS. He and his fellow bishops who worked to reform Vatican policy were not asking for a reversal of *Humanae Vitae*. That move could have spelled disaster given the theological climate in Rome at the time; there was no tolerance for diversity on the birth control issue. They simply asked the church to agree that using a condom to prevent AIDS was the lesser of two evils and a way to save lives. For this action Dowling was rebuked at least twice by the South African papal nuncio because he was not following Vatican policy.[8]

Apparently, to get the church back on track and to reiterate its position on condoms and AIDS, a prominent member of the Roman Curia, Cardinal Alfonso Trujillo, declared that the use of condoms is morally wrong. As president of the Vatican's Pontifical Council for the Family, he undoubtedly had the support of the pope in stating without reservation in 2003 that the church's ban on condoms was absolute.[9] The use of condoms to prevent AIDS was therefore unacceptable, he said. In seeking to emphasize his point, Trujillo claimed that the HIV virus could pass through the latex condom and thus it offered little or no protection against the disease. This marked the first time Vatican officials asserted that condoms were ineffective, and therefore, why would anyone want to use them? The use of condoms was immoral *and* ineffective.

The World Health Organization (WHO) and numerous scientists declared this statement to be totally false and demanded that the Vatican withdraw it immediately. Dr. Catherine Hankins, chief scientific advisor to UNAIDS, responded that Trujillo's statements "are totally incorrect. Latex condoms are impermeable. They do prevent HIV transmission."[10] Nevertheless, Catholic leaders remained steadfast in their position and did not admit they were wrong. The campaign against condoms had reached a new level of ecclesiastical spin. The cardinal ignored scientifically demonstrated facts to promote church doctrine, and never admitted his error. Trujillo stayed on the job and the church had egg on its face.

This leads us to two important points about organizational theory and change. First, many scholars pay little attention to deviant behavior by organizational incumbents.[11] In order to maintain the status quo, incumbents in the Catholic Church and elsewhere present disingenuous ideas to maintain their hold on power and their view of the organization's normative system. In other words, they lie. Bishops and cardinals sprinkle a little holy water on the conflict and move on. In the period of conflict and argumentation we should expect this kind of behavior from both sides and watch for it. Second, the Trujillo statement uncovers a new field of interest—medical science; this group entered the church discussion and supported the views of challengers. This is called a "distant" field in organizational analysis because it joins the conflict after the fight already started. A distant field (viz., medical science) can help or hinder the quest for social change in an organization; in this case it acts as an advocate for change. As Trujillo's comments suggest, the Catholic Church and its Vatican officials did not play by the rules. When confronted with irrefutable evidence, we would expect losers to acknowledge defeat and move on. We find in this study that high ranking church officials maintained irrational views of reality, while simultaneously ignoring the possibility that loyal Catholics could very well suffer and die as a result of such misrepresentations. Why did the church fail to correct its error? UNAIDS and many others would certainly like to know. Trujillo died in 2008, and so we will never know why he took such an erroneous position regarding condoms and AIDS.[12]

Fortunately, some important Catholic scholars saw what was going on and reflected seriously on these issues; they tried to clarify the more important points in the discussion. Popes and bishops were debating ethical issues, and so it was time for moral theologians to respond. In 2004, Fr. Martin Rhonheimer wrote a review essay in *The Tablet* which provided both sides food for thought. As a consultant attached to the Congregation for the Doctrine of the Faith (CDF), his views held considerable weight in the world of bishops and cardinals. Of course, we would expect him to say that he fully supported the teachings of *Humanae Vitae* since he consulted for CDF. One does not get jobs like that by being a dissident regarding papal teachings. In his essay, Rhonheimer stated that he was opposed to the use of artificial birth control and rejected the contraceptive mentality. But he offered some important distinctions as he plowed through years of commentary on the norms of Catholic married life. He then asserted that condoms cannot be considered intrinsically evil; only human acts get that label, not things. When discussing persons who have HIV, he writes, that "the moral norm condemning contraception as intrinsically evil does not apply in these cases."[13] What then, is the path to follow?

First he stresses the importance of abstinence and fidelity for all Catholics; they should live a well-ordered sexual life. He does not formally ban the use of condoms for a person who has AIDS (two popes did), but Rhonheimer stresses that he assumes the people he counsels will act with a sense of responsibility. When dealing with sexually promiscuous individuals, for example prostitutes, he claims that their use of condoms "will help to reduce the evil consequences of morally evil behavior."[14] Moreover, it is his belief that the church cannot possibly teach that people who engage in immoral lifestyles should avoid using condoms. For 2004, these ideas proved to be a major breakthrough and turned a few heads at the Vatican. No one at the higher levels of Catholic institutional thinking condemned him for writing this article. The essay in *The Tablet* was allowed to stand on its own merits. He did, however, received criticism from ultra-conservative Catholics who march to the beat of their own drummer. In retrospect one can see that Rhonheimer's ideas, which were articulated in 2004, fit in nicely with the U.S. bishops' statement (1987), the education plan of Austria's archbishop (1995), and the statements of Bishop Dowling from South Africa (2001). Nonetheless, the church was not ready to embrace these notions in the 1980s and 1990s. This slowness to act harmed many people throughout the world. Martin Rhonheimer, a well-known member of *Opus Dei*, was allowed to speak his mind without penalty in the twenty-first century. He was not rebuked by any papal nuncio. Was the church beginning to change its views on condoms and AIDS as Pope John Paul II was about to die? The wheels of change turn ever so slowly in Rome.

It is evident from this discussion that the *dead zone* created by *Veritatis Splendor* had evaporated by 2002 and bishops and theologians were talking openly and debating whether condoms could be used to prevent the spread of AIDS. Nevertheless, much time had been lost in this crucial battle to fight AIDS. On the positive side, a bishop from South Africa had entered the discussion, and his pastoral experience seemed to trump assertions of curial canon lawyers. Why not listen to the man who has walked in clinics and given communion to those dying of AIDS? Isn't he the most credible witness in the church about moral and ethical norms concerning AIDS? The debate continued in the Catholic Church with no resolution in sight. Was there any hope for change at the papal apartments? Only time would tell.

NOTES

1. See National Catholic Register, 2007; www.ncregister.com/site/article/africas_catholic_explosion/ (accessed December 6, 2012).
2. Helen Epstein, *The Invisible Cure* (New York: Farrar, Strauss, 2007), 46.
3. Marcella Alsan, "The Church & AIDS in Africa: Condoms & the Culture of Life," *Commonweal*, April 17, 2006, 24.
4. "AIDS Conference in Vienna with Call for More Funding," July 19, 2010; www.caritas.org/activities/hiv_aids/CompassionForPeopleLivingWithAids.html (accessed January 12, 2012).

5. Raymond Copson, "CRS Issue Brief for Congress: AIDS in Africa," Catholic Relief Services, Washington, D.C., May 28, 2004.

6. Peter Piot, *No Time to Lose* (New York, Norton, 2012), 56.

7. "Condoms for Catholics?" *Newsweek*, July 20, 2001, 24.

8. Personal Interview with Bishop Kevin Dowling, Notre Dame University, March 28, 2012.

9. Alfonso Trujillo, "Family Values versus Safe Sex," Paper of the Pontifical Council for the Family, December 1, 2003.

10. Quoted in BBC NEWS October 9, 2003; http://news.bbc.co.uk/2/hi/health/3176982.stm; of course, nothing human is perfect; condoms prove to be 2 percent defective according to U.S. studies.

11. Neil Fligstein and Doug McAdam, "Toward a General Theory of Strategic Action Fields," *Sociological Theory* 29, no. 1 (2011): 23.

12. One charitable explanation is that Trujillo heard that lamb skin condoms have small pores which may allow the HIV virus to pass through; hence medical experts tell people they should use latex condoms, not lamb skin. The cardinal may have over-generalized.

13. Martin Rhonheimer, "The Truth about Condoms," *The Tablet*, July 10, 2004, 12.

14. Rhonheimer, "The Truth about Condoms," 13.

6

+

New Voices from Other Altars

Whenever I think of the word "bishop" my mind invariably turns to the idea of "cathedral" since that is where a bishop works, prays, ordains, and preaches. Of course, a central focus of the bishop's diocese—the cathedral—is the altar where Mass is celebrated daily. There we will find his chair, which is a symbol of his teaching office. It is from these sacred places that a new message about alleviating human pain and suffering went forth. After South Africa's Bishop Dowling challenged Vatican leaders to change their teaching about condoms and AIDS, there emerged a huge echo in other cathedrals which reverberated around the globe. Fellow bishops began to speak out in support of the South African bishop's proposal. With over 30 million people—men, women, and children—living with HIV/AIDS by the year 2000,[1] some high ranking church officials probably were wondering if they were doing enough to prevent the spread of HIV/AIDS.

In 2004 Bishop Juan Camino, the general secretary of Spain's Conference of Catholic Bishops, informed the religious and secular media that there should be a place in church moral theology for the use of condoms to prevent the spread of AIDS. "Condoms have a place," he said, "in the global prevention of AIDS."[2] A small group of his supporters agreed and asked the Vatican to change. Opposition to Vatican policy was duly noted, and Rome quickly applied pressure to squelch dissent. It was 1987 (United States) and 1996 (Austria) all over again. The full body of Spain's conference of bishops rejected the ideas of this reformist group and sided with the pope. The Spanish bishops officially went on record saying that the "use of contraceptives implies immoral sexual behavior." They explained that it is "not true that the church has changed its doctrine on condoms," adding, "it's impossible to advise the use of condoms" under Catholic doctrine.[3]

Even the casual observer of Catholic life could readily see that a church social movement was beginning to take shape, despite the fact that powerful forces within the Vatican wanted to put a stop to it. This social movement to address the AIDS conundrum was not led by the liberal laity or disgruntled deacons, but rather by a band of brave bishops. All was not well in the papal apartments, and many outside Vatican City felt that a policy change might be in order. In fact, opposition forces took a crucial step toward church reform: they decided to go public and draw media attention. All the elements needed for a strong social movement were beginning to fall into place, at least according to one leading social change theory articulated by John McCarthy and Mayer Zald.[4] These pioneers of sociological theory bring to bear classic insights that have had lasting influence on the study of organizations and change. They argued that a social movement needs strong and powerful leaders to confront the status quo, if it is to succeed. Skilled actors must mobilize the target population; there must be a coalescence of individual groups working for change. Moreover, the media will become useful in communicating key ideas.

By using the historical-case-study method we have been able to uncover a key component of church reform, and it is a social movement headed by high ranking church officials (skillful actors), who use the social media. They demonstrate cognitive skills, empathetic approaches toward those who suffer, and high level communication skills. Fligstein and McAdam underscore the importance of these factors when they state "that actors who undertake strategic action must be able to use whatever perspective they have developed in an intersubjective enough fashion to secure the willing cooperation of others."[5] This new movement in the church would continue to gain new followers, expand, and prosper.

A few months after the pullback by the full body of Spain's conference of bishops, Felipe Arizmendi, bishop of San Cristobal, Mexico, presented his ideas to the press. In late 2004 he said that condom use to prevent AIDS was a lesser evil when compared to the spread of AIDS, and that people have an obligation not to infect others.[6] Then, in a move that surprised papal insiders, the reformists gained coalescence when Cardinal Georges Cottier, the theologian to the pontifical household in Rome, joined the progressives and stated that change was needed. He made these comments no more than one hundred yards from the papal apartments. The movement for a new church policy gained momentum when he joined the dissidents who argued that church policy must be revised. Note, there clearly was a church policy at this time, and certain bishops asked that it be changed. Cottier told the Italian press in February 2005, that in his view condoms could be used by a married couple, but only for the purpose of preventing the spread of HIV/AIDS.[7] Thus, those at the highest level of the Roman Catholic Church bureaucracy were voicing their opposition to a long-standing papal teaching. Cardinals and bishops were reading the "signs of the times,"[8] and then taking action.

These bishops were following a traditional approach to church reform when (1) they acknowledged that the pope and legitimate councils teach authentic Catholic doctrine, unless it is withdrawn or rejected by subsequent popes or councils. Hence, (2) when conflict arises, bishops must ask the pope to reconsider his ideas in light of their pastoral insights and suggestions. They do this (3) by telling the pope why they think he is in error. With John Paul II ailing and near death due to complications of Parkinson's disease (2003–2005), a sense of church dysfunction arose and top leaders saw the need to speak out in order to save lives. The Vatican was in no mood to respond to these challenges, given that the pope was dying. Yet, everyone realized important decisions still had to be made.

This two decade stalemate is reminiscent of Charles Kimball's discussion of dysfunctional religion in the modern era. He sums up the issue rather well: "Religious world views and inflexible doctrines among Christian groups have often presented serious problems in the face of scientific inquiries and hypotheses."[9] Top officials in the Catholic Church stood fast in their opposition to using condoms to fight the spread of HIV/AIDS. In contrast, Dr. Koop and a host of medical experts advocated a program of abstinence, fidelity, *and condoms* to save lives. Many bishops asked the pope to reconsider his position, but theological paralysis had already set in.

Kimball continues his discussion of religion as a social problem by pointing out two major warning signs of dysfunctional religion: (1) absolute truth claims by religious leaders and (2) blind obedience.[10] Of course, all religions make truth claims, but Kimball states that he is concerned when human leaders interpret these claims as "propositions requiring uniform assent and are treated as rigid doctrines." When this happens the "likelihood of corruption in that tradition rises exponentially."[11] Almost all the cardinals and bishops who objected to the pope's stance about condoms were rebuffed. They were told to get in line with the papal program without further discussion. The topic was never brought up for serious discussion during numerous synods held in Rome during twenty years of public debate regarding AIDS. The 1989 meeting in Rome about AIDS simply reiterated papal pronouncements. On this particular issue, the church was clearly dysfunctional: it could not solve its theological or public policy problems as demonstrated by the fact that bishops kept saying popes were wrong and they had to change. Popes, on the other hand, rejected these suggestions. As one of my old professors used to say when frustrated by inept university administrators, "John, that's no way to run a railroad." We might add, "That is no way to run a church." And many Catholics died of AIDS during this period of stonewalling by Vatican officials.

What bishops and cardinals were doing in the twenty-first century was similar to what happened during the time of St. Augustine. The fifth-century bishop of Hippo joined other bishops of North Africa and confronted Pope Zosimus about his support of Pelagius, a heretic according to the Council of Carthage (412 AD). The corpulent monk from Britain had persuaded the pope that his teachings did not deny the fallen nature of man nor the role of grace in performing virtuous acts. Augustine and his colleagues had it all wrong. With opposition from North Africa growing and the emperor peeved at conflict in the provinces, the bishop of Rome wrote his famous *Epistola Tractoria* (418), condemning Pelagius, as the North African bishops had done previously. The pope changed his views when confronted by the arguments of his fellow bishops. Augustine and his colleagues challenged the pope and saved the church from heresy.[12]

We should note that history records no one ever died of Pelagianism. AIDS was killing people left and right and the church stood its ground: just before he died of complications from Parkinson's disease, Pope John Paul II urged abstinence and fidelity to reduce the spread of AIDS. He had again rejected the use of condoms to prevent AIDS. Two decades of criticism and confrontation apparently had little effect on this authoritarian pope.[13] It is worth noting that one of the side effects of Parkinson's disease is rigid thinking.[14] Nevertheless, the strength of the pope's claim to absolute truth and blind obedience was beginning to erode. Many church officials were questioning the Vatican's condoms/AIDS policy, and opposition forces were growing. Not all bishops were willing to follow the papal call to arms and maintain the status quo. The new pope would have his work cut out as John Paul II breathed his last on April 2, 2005. In many respects he was a great man and his spiritual legacy will be remembered for years to come; but in the end conservative ideology got the best of him.

NOTES

1. Kaiser Family Foundation, "The Global HIV/AIDS Epidemic," *Fact Sheet*, June, 2001.

2. Austen Ivereigh, "Towards a New Morality: Condoms and Church Teaching," *The Tablet* (November 27, 2010). Also read: Associated Press, "Spain's Catholic Church Reverses Statement in Support of Condom Use to Prevent AIDS," January 20, 2005.

3. Spanish bishops react: www.lifesitenews.com/news/archive/ldn/1950/dec/5012005 (accessed December 28, 2012). Also see D. Williams, "Spanish Bishops," *Washington Post*, January 20, 2005.

4. John McCarthy and Mayer Zald, "Resource Mobilization and Social Movements," *American Journal of Sociology* 82 (1977): 1225.

5. Neil Fligstein and Doug McAdam, "Toward a General Theory of Strategic Action Fields," *Sociological Theory* 29 (2011): 7

6. Laurence Iliff, "Mexican Bishop Backs Condom Use," *Dallas Morning News*, January 21, 2005. Review of previous statements on condoms and AIDS.

7. Sophie Arie, "Cardinal Says Condoms Could Help to Stop AIDS," *The Guardian (UK)*, February 1, 2005.

8. See *Gaudium and Spes*, Vatican II, 1965. Well known phrase used often in the document *Church in the Modern World*.

9. Charles Kimball, *When Religion Becomes Evil* (New York: HarperCollins, 2002), 29.

10. Kimball, *When Religion*, 41–99.

11. Kimball, *When Religion*, 50.

12. Henry Chadwick, *The Early Church* (New York: Penquin, 1993), 231; see also William Jurgens, *The Faith of the Early Fathers* 2 (Collegeville, MN: Liturgical Press, 1979), 214.

13. Alan Riding, "Theologians in Europe Challenge Pope's Conservative Leadership," *New York Times*, July 14, 1989. See the Cologne Declaration, 1989.

14. Patrick McNamara et al., "Dopaminergic Syndromes," *Sleep and Hypnosis* 4, no. 3 (2002): 119–31; www.bu.edu/phylogeny/publications/Dopamine%20and%20sleep%20from%20S&H.pdf (accessed February 23, 2013).

7

+

New Pope

Chance for Change

With the funeral ceremonies for John Paul II completed on April 8, 2005, preparations began in earnest for the election of a new pope. The church must go on. News stories continued to pour in about the spiritual legacy of the Polish Pope; a great leader had passed. He would be a tough act to follow, and, as *Time* magazine's man of the year in 1994, he was one of the most recognizable faces on the planet. The last five years of his life were filled with pain and suffering due to various illnesses. Having examined John Paul in 2000, a U.S. neurologist, Dr. Vincent Fortanasce, recently revealed some new details about the pope's condition five years before his death.[1] The physician happened to be vacationing in Italy and decided to attend a Mass celebrated by the pontiff in August 2000. He thought that Pope John Paul appeared rather frail; he needed a cane to move around the altar. Dr. Fortanasce volunteered his services to Vatican officials, and within a few days he examined and treated John Paul for about thirty minutes. At that time the pope was diagnosed with a severe cervical problem and difficulties with motor coordination (shuffling gait), and was clearly suffering from "moderately advanced" Parkinson's disease. The last few years of his life were difficult. Now the church had to find his successor.

Many cardinals were already in Rome for the pope's funeral, and once all 115 had finally arrived, the conclave could begin as scheduled: April 18, 2005. There were technically 117 voting members (all cardinals under eighty years of age) called to the conclave, but two cardinals could not attend due to health issues. All but 3 of the 117 voting members were appointed by John Paul II during his twenty-seven-year reign as Roman pontiff.[2] Thus his influence over church affairs would continue long after his death. Rumors swirled throughout the Vatican about who were the favorites to become the next pope (*papabile*), but insiders cautioned, "He who goes in the conclave a pope, comes out a cardinal." Speculation centered on three prominent candidates: Joseph Ratzinger, prefect of the Congregation for the Doctrine of the Faith, Cardinal Jorge Bergoglio of Argentina, and Cardinal Carlo Martini, retired archbishop of Milan. If those rumors had any validity, they would indicate that participants in the conclave were looking both inside and outside Italy for a new pope.[3]

The conclave itself took place in the Sistine Chapel, but after deliberations and voting the cardinals resided in the newly constructed St. Martha's House (Domus Sanctae Marthae), which is a short walk from the hall with the famous ceiling painted by Michelangelo. Complete secrecy is the rule for all conclaves, but somehow information about papal elections always manages to reach the anxious public. During this conclave's early voting rounds, one needed a two-thirds majority to become pope (seventy-seven votes). After the first ballot, the traditional white smoke did not rise from the Sistine Chapel's famous chimney. More discussion and balloting would be needed to select the second pope of the twenty-first century. On the fourth ballot, Cardinal Joseph Ratzinger was selected as the new pontiff, and he chose the name Benedict XVI for his time as pope and bishop of Rome. On April 19, 2005, Benedict took over the reins of a church in turmoil due to the priest sex-abuse scandal and other pressing issues, including the church's AIDS policy.

Joseph Ratzinger was now the head of the 1.2 billion member Roman Catholic Church, with four hundred thousand priests, and was no stranger to informed Vatican observers. He arrived at Vatican City in 1981 from his native Germany at the behest of John Paul II to become the prefect of the Congregation for the Doctrine of the Faith. For twenty-five years he was the "enforcer" of Catholic orthodoxy, and the job probably put him on many enemy lists around the ecclesiastical world. Joseph was born in 1927, and by the late 1930s he dreamed of becoming a priest, but the road to the seminary had to go through Hitler's Third Reich. At fourteen he joined "Hitler Youth," which was required of all young men in those days, but he never attended meetings. His father was anti-Nazi. Joseph was later drafted out of the seminary in 1943 and served his Nazi superiors as an anti-aircraft specialist until the end of the war in 1945 when he ended up in a POW camp. Although he is the only pope we know of who, as a young man, uttered the infamous words "Heil Hitler"—a requirement when any Nazi officer entered a room—he was never a member of the Nazi political party. Like many combatants who were judged to be "doing their duty" by serving in the German army, he was released by the Allied Forces, returned home, and reenrolled in the local seminary to prepare for the priesthood. Joseph Ratzinger was ordained in 1951 and went on for higher doctoral studies where he specialized in the works of Augustine, Aquinas, and Bonaventure. He was judged to be an outstanding scholar in his early thirties, and so it was no surprise that Cardinal Joseph Frings of Cologne named him as his peritus (expert) at the Second Vatican Council (1962–1965). At first he embraced the progressive movement in the church started by Pope John XXIII and counted liberal theologians Edward Schillebeeckx, Yves Congar, and Karl Rahner as his mentors. Due to their controversial theological stands, all three had been sanctioned by the Holy Office (read: Ottaviani) before the council even began. Later experiences while teaching at the University of Tübingen and pastoral work counseling university students led Joseph to distrust some of the directions the church and society were headed. Gradually he began to question some of the social movements for change in and outside the church. He left teaching and quickly rose through the ecclesiastical ranks to become archbishop of Munich and then cardinal in 1977. He was among the last group of bishops that Paul VI named in a consistory to be cardinals before his death in 1978. He supported the pope's encyclical *Humanae Vitae*, unlike many leading bishops in Europe who had grave misgivings about the papal ban on birth control. Ratzinger gradually moved away from the 1960s progressive theology developed at Vatican II, and by the time he officiated at the funeral of John Paul II, everyone knew he had become a theological conservative: he (1) opposed the notion of a married clergy, (2) objected to the idea of liberation theology, (3) rejected the concept of women priests, (4) favored the program to allow conservative Catholics the right to celebrate Mass said in Latin and of course, (5) asserted that artificial birth control was immoral and condoms could not be used to prevent AIDS. When he was elected pope at age seventy-eight, his pastoral experience during the previous twenty-five years was nil.

Despite his curial resume and Nazi background, some leaders in the Catholic Church and many in the scientific community were looking to him for a change in Catholic health care policy. AIDS workers were hopeful that "there may be room for maneuver when it comes to the new Pope's position on condom use."[4] Many Catholics within the church had similar views. Yet, in a June 2005 speech to African bishops, the new pope stated that the "spread of HIV and AIDS in Africa should be tackled through fidelity and abstinence and not by condoms."[5] There was nothing new here; he was following the line of the previous administration which he had been supporting for two decades. But many found this stance hard to fathom since African public health studies revealed that by 2005, 30 percent of pregnant women in South Africa were infected with HIV; this amounted to about ten million expectant mothers.[6] More had to be done to prevent the spread of AIDS, according to church reformers. The new pope had officially joined the "Catholic Party of NO" in his speech to African bishops. All hopes that Pope Benedict would inaugurate a new program to fight the spread of AIDS were quickly dashed by the Rock of St. Peter.

Nonetheless, the voices of opposition around the world grew louder. Their tactics were clear: speak out and use the media to let Vatican officials know they were on the wrong track. In the fall of 2005 Bishop Kevin Dowling of South Africa once again asked the Vatican to change its stand on the use of condoms to prevent the spread of AIDS. He stated that the church ban on the use of condoms to prevent the spread of AIDS was morally unacceptable.[7]

Not to be outdone in theological insights, Cardinal Javier Barragán, then president of the Pontifical Council for the Pastoral Care of Health Care Workers, weighed in; the pope must change, he said. It became clear that the social movement for change in the church was gaining momentum. But when I asked Bishop Kevin Dowling if anyone was coordinating these news conferences, he informed me that to his knowledge all episcopal statements arose due to their own personal convictions on how to respond to the AIDS crisis.[8] No one was coordinating their statements to the media. In 2006 Barragán asserted that condoms could be used in certain circumstances, such as "when a woman cannot refuse her HIV-positive husband's sexual advances."[9] Several other bishops and cardinals at this time argued that one must use a condom if he or she has AIDS in order to obey the commandment "Thou shalt not kill" (Deut 5:17). The laity and some journalists quickly joined forces with the bishops. Marcella Alsan, MD, a woman physician who had worked extensively in African Catholic hospitals, wrote that the church's opposition to the use of condoms "may mean not only untold human suffering, but the loss of millions of human lives."[10] Why this dark view of church policy? She is a doctor and trained in the science of medicine. Doctors routinely tell their patients that if they have a sexually transmitted disease, they should use a condom when having sex. That makes eminent medical sense.

Reflecting many of the same concerns expressed by Alsan, Nicholas Kristof of the *New York Times* wrote that in "Zimbabwe, I visited a Catholic charity that gave out condoms—until the bishop found out." Kristof is convinced that "the Vatican's ban on condoms has cost many hundreds of thousands of lives from AIDS."[11] Strong words from a Pulitzer Prize–winning reporter who has written on several global health issues. One can see why numerous bishops sought to change Vatican policy; they wanted to save lives and join the world community in the fight against AIDS. Nevertheless, the institutional Catholic Church maintained its traditional moral stand while at the same time many pointed out that this rigid stance was killing people.

The tipping point in the debate came in April 2006 when seventy-nine-year-old Cardinal Carlo Martini, retired archbishop of Milan, entered the fray. In an interview with the Italian magazine *l'Espresso* he stated that the Vatican should allow the use of condoms for married couples if one partner is infected with the HIV / AIDS virus.[12] It is a "lesser evil," he said. The key point that apparently caught the Vatican's attention was the well-publicized report that many monogamous Catholic married women were being infected with AIDS by their promiscuous husbands. They were faithful, but what good was that doing them? Thus, women should be allowed to protect themselves from HIV and not be forced to have unprotected sex with their husbands—an act that ultimately could leave their children orphans. Bishops were now using the argument of self-defense to push for a new church policy. Surprisingly, the Vatican blinked. Within a week of Martini's remarks, Pope Benedict established a commission of Catholic scholars to look into the condom controversy.[13] Finally, the social movement to bring about change had a victory. The group had shown itself to be a legitimate "field" in sociological theory because it had a significant effect on church policy. The pope responded. The Vatican could no longer make pronouncements and expect people to follow. A document about this commission's findings would be released soon, according to Vatican insiders. The powerful Cardinal Martini, who had received a significant number of votes to be pope at the 2005 conclave, had many friends at the highest levels of church bureaucracy. The pressure on Pope Benedict must have been enormous. The challengers had won a small victory. The waiting game to hear about the findings of the newly established Vatican commission was the next hurdle to be overcome.

NOTES

1. Robert Pool, "Arcadia Doctor Recalls Consultation with Pope John Paul II," *L.A. Times*, December 31, 2011.
2. John Rivera and Mike Leary, "Pope John Paul II Dies," *Baltimore Sun*, April 3, 2005; also see www.catholicnews.com / jpii / stories / concl06.htm (accessed March 6, 2012).
3. John Allen, "Profile: New Pope, Jesuit Bergoglio, Was Runner-Up in 2005 Conclave," *National Catholic Reporter*, March 3, 2013.
4. Declan Butler, "Conclave Kindles Hope for Bioethical Reform," *Nature* 434 (April 21, 2005), 944.
5. "Pope Rejects Condoms for Africa"; quoted from BBC News, June 10, 2005; see http: / / news.bbc.co.uk / 2 / hi / europe / 4081276.stm (accessed March 6, 2013).
6. Mark Cichocki, "HIV around the World—South Africa," February 11, 2011; http: / / aids.about.com / od / clinicaltrials / a / safrica_2.htm (accessed May 4, 2013).

7. Laurie Goering, "South African Bishop Bucks the Vatican," *Chicago Tribune*, November 4, 2005.

8. Interview with Bishop Kevin Dowling, Notre Dame University, March 28, 2012.

9. "Vatican Studying Condoms and AIDS," www.usatoday.com/news/world/2006-04-25-vatican-condoms_x.htm (accessed March 6, 2012).

10. Marcella Alsan, "The Church and AIDS in Africa: Condoms and the Culture of Life," *Commonweal*, April 24, 2006, 12.

11. Nicholas Kristof, "The Pope and AIDS," *New York Times*, May 8, 2005.

12. Cardinal Martini statement: www.msnbc.msn.com/id/12424425/ns/world_news-europe/ (accessed February 22, 2011).

13. F. Gray, "Vatican to Rule on AIDS and Condoms," *CatholicHerald.co.uk*, April 28, 2006, 1.

8

Waiting for Godot

The Lost Years

Benedict XVI barely had time to clear out his desk at the curia and move his grand piano into the papal apartments when forces within and outside the church began asking for changes in church policy. The church had been at a standstill for the previous few years because John Paul was weak and unable to work with colleagues on numerous pressing issues. Fiona Ehlers writes: "Events and personnel decisions had been postponed during his [John Paul II] last few years, in which he was ill. The new pope was expected to finally clear off the desks and give the Curia a fresh start."[1] Already in 2001 Peter Piot, executive director of UNAIDS, made this observation about church policy: "When priests preach against using contraception [to prevent AIDS], they are committing a serious mistake which is costing human lives. We do not ask the church to promote contraception, but merely to stop banning its use."[2] Dr. Piot—himself a Catholic—simply wanted the church to cooperate with health care experts in the A+B+C plan, which included the use of condoms to prevent the spread of AIDS. There had been no real dialogue on this point in the John Paul II era, however. For the new pope, health care and AIDS had to become a top priority. Since the first cases of acquired immune deficiency syndrome were reported in 1981, worldwide HIV infections had grown to pandemic proportions.[3] With an estimated 33.3 million people throughout the world infected with HIV by 2005 (see figure 8.1), and about 8 percent of them children, health care professionals were looking for help from all sectors, including the Vatican.[4] On the twenty-fifth anniversary of the AIDS epidemic, Dr. Anthony Fauci put the situation succinctly, "With 4.3 million new HIV infections each year throughout the world, we

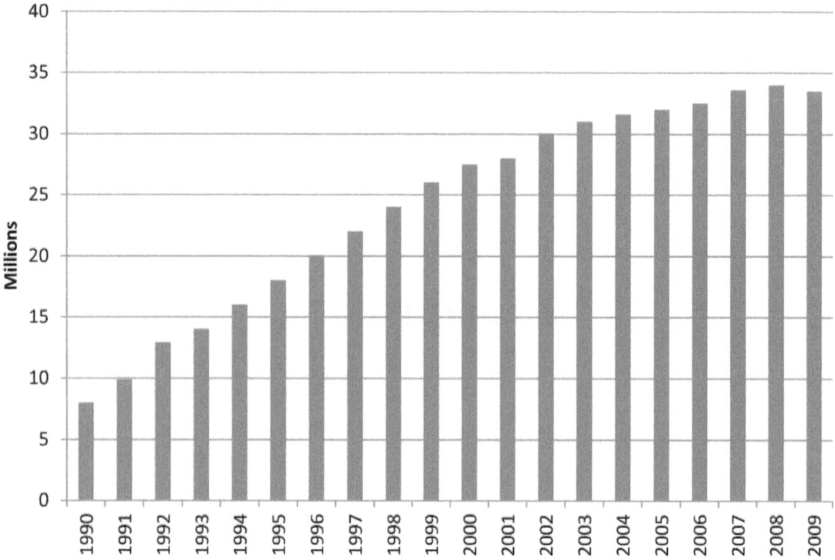

Figure 8.1. Global Numbers of People Living with HIV, by Year. UNAIDS, Global Report, 2010.

face an untenable situation, as new HIV infections far outstrip our ability to treat all those infected."[5] The reformist clerics calling for more effective action by the Catholic Church appeared to be on the right track, according to Piot and Fauci. Something had to be done since HIV infections had tripled since 1990, and Pope Benedict was facing a full-court press by colleagues asking for change. He had ordered a comprehensive study on the church's position on condoms and AIDS, but no final decision had been reached by 2007 about lifting the ban on condoms.

In a 2010 article for the Jesuit journal, *The Tablet,* Austen Ivereigh reported that in April 2006, Cardinal Javier Lozano Barragán invited moral theologians and other scholars to submit papers to his council on "the use of condoms by those with AIDS." Barragán went on to state that "my council is studying this attentively with scientists and theologians expressly charged with preparing a document on the subject, which will be made public soon."[6] Another year passed and no report was issued by the Vatican on the condoms/AIDS issue. Complete secrecy was the standard in such church matters, and it is only through the efforts of Austen Ivereigh and his Vatican contacts that we are now able to piece together the twists and turns of Vatican bureaucracy at the highest level. Ivereigh writes, "In 2008, while at a conference in Rome, I happened to meet a senior CDF official (I won't give his name) and asked him what had happened to the commission [report]."[7] The answer to this simple inquiry is astounding, as we will see.

Between 2006 and 2007 Cardinal Javier Lozano Barragán, president of the Pontifical Council for Health Care, prepared a 200-page dossier on whether it is legitimate for Catholics to use condoms to protect someone from contracting HIV/AIDS. This report was subsequently sent to the Congregation for the Doctrine of the Faith for review and publication. One of the key conclusions of the report was the recommendation that church teaching should espouse the principle that it is morally preferable for an HIV infected man/woman to use a condom rather than not use one. The crucial issue, as Ivereigh writes was "whether it is morally preferable for an infected man to use a condom than not to use one. The consensus of moral theologians—and this was doubtless reflected in Cardinal Lozano Barragán's report—is a firm YES."[8]

The CDF studied the report and its findings, but decided to shelve the report since accepting and releasing it would cause a Catholic PR problem. According to Ivereigh, church leaders at CDF took the position that there was no way they could go public with the report without being misunderstood.[9] Change would be confusing to the faithful, and CDF feared headlines in the newspapers like "Pope Backs Use of Condoms." Thus, nothing was going to be published on the subject; Pope Benedict certainly had to approve of this strategy. The church was not going to take a stand which could have saved lives. A group of highly motivated bishops over a period of twenty years asked for a change; Barragán's commission recommended change; but the CDF and the pope said "no."

What is clear to anyone who reviews the literature on suppressing Barragán's report is that no mention is made about those who are at risk of getting AIDS and whether a policy is in place to save lives. Officials at CDF were concerned about the church's image. All discussion was about how the church would look if its teachings were altered. Little wonder why Ivereigh concludes his review of this episode on contemporary church history with this scathing comment:

> By choosing not to say anything—and by burying the report—the Church remains vulnerable to the accusation that its teaching on this point is inhumane and irrational. But even worse is the deliberate suppression of theological truth for fear of being misunderstood. It is mundane. It is cowardly. It is not worthy of a teaching authority which proclaims that the truth sets us free.[10]

Bishops and others who were critical of the church's stand on this point felt constrained to keep silent since the pope had ordered a study on the matter. The feeling was: let them research the topic and see what they come up with. If there were flaws in their arguments and conclusions, there would be time for an appropriate response. Unfortunately, what this papal call for research did accomplish *de facto* was to create another "dead zone." There was little or no activity by challengers to change the policy in question while waiting for the report. Like the two men in Samuel Beckett's play *Waiting for Godot*, nothing happened despite the promise of a special visitor.

The previous dead zone in this twenty-year-old debate emerged earlier when Pope John Paul issued his 1993 encyclical *Veritatis Splendor* wherein he declared that the use of condoms was intrinsically evil. In 2001, someone did break the silence caused by the papal letter and asked for a change in AIDS policy. Yes, that person was Bishop Dowling of South Africa. Due to these organizational dead zones, fully ten years of possible social change, discussion, and progress were thwarted. The Vatican has subtle and not so subtle ways of keeping people quiet. Two popes failed to respond effectively to a crucial social problem and thousands of AIDS patients died while others acquired the disease during this period of inaction. That was religious malpractice. This is not to say that Catholics stood by and did nothing. As noted previously, about 25 percent of the care AIDS victims receive worldwide is provided by Catholic organizations, but the church had a chance to play an even more important role in preventing the spread of a dreadful disease. It failed to do so.

In summary, I feel it is important that we remind ourselves what has just been covered thus far:

1. Cardinals and bishops were arguing about the papal stand on condoms and AIDS. Some were for change and others not.
2. The pope said he would appoint a commission to study the matter. [Does this sound like déjà vu all over again, e.g., the birth control commission?]
3. After an extensive study and the production of a 200-page report, the experts on the committee apparently told the pope to change policy on banning condoms so as to save lives. Do the right thing and tell people to use a condom if they have HIV / AIDS.
4. Church officials at CDF said they could not make the report public because the Vatican would be misunderstood.
5. The Catholic Church decides to do nothing and does not even tell the public that the Barragán report would not be released.

This is no way for a religious group to deal with a modern social problem. But now we have come close to understanding the nature of "paralysis" in the church; because of many deeply held cultural norms and values, no one at the top of the ecclesiastical pyramid could move in the direction recommended by local pastors. Church leaders were asked to change by subordinates who were on the front lines fighting AIDS, but they did nothing. This issue is not a "hot button" topic like women's ordination, the priest sexual-abuse crisis, or married priests. The crucial point had to do with medical ethics and saving lives; the top leadership of the church was unable to move in the right direction. Little wonder why Garry Wills calls this Vatican blunder one of the greatest scandals in contemporary church history. "More people are more resentful and hateful toward the Catholic Church because of that [condoms and AIDS] than because of the sexual molestation problem . . . but for the most part they did not kill people. This is killing people on a grand scale, and it's a horrendous scandal, much greater than any sexual molestation scandal."[11] By putting Catholics at risk for contracting HIV/AIDS through its no-condoms-for-prevention policy, many church members died and spread the disease to others rather than committing the sin of disobedience. Peter Piot, Dr. Marcella Alsan, and Nick Kristof said as much. How can popes celebrate Mass at St. Peter's Square and then go to bed at night with a clear conscience? We will answer that question later.

NOTES

1. Fiona Ehlers et al., "Exhausted in the Vatican: The Final Battles of Pope Benedict XVI," *Der Spiegel*, June 15, 2012.
2. Peter Piot as quoted in "Church's Stand against Contraception Costs Lives," *Agence France Presse*, June 29, 2001.
3. Pandemics are infectious disease epidemics that are widespread and literally jump continents.
4. Joint United Nations Programme on HIV/AIDS 2010 (UNAIDS), "Global Report." Also see: "Report on the Global AIDS Epidemic," Geneva, Switzerland: UNAIDS, 2006.
5. Anthony Fauci, "Twenty-Five Years of HIV/AIDS," May 25, 2007; www.project-syndicate.org/commentary/twenty-five-years-of-hiv-aids (accessed June 22, 2013).
6. Austen Ivereigh, "Towards a New Morality: Condoms and Church Teaching," *The Tablet* (November 27, 2010), www.thetablet.co.uk/article/15577 (accessed February 2, 2012).
7. Austen Ivereigh, "Pope on Condoms and AIDS," *America* (November 21, 2010).
8. Austen Ivereigh, "AIDS, Condoms, and the Suppression of Theological Truth," *America* (February 11, 2010), 23.
9. Ivereigh, "AIDS, Condoms, 25.
10. Ivereigh, "AIDS, Condoms," 27.
11. Amy Welborn interview with Garry Wills; http://amywelborn.typepad.com/openbook/2006/03/pope_garry.html (accessed May 31, 2012).

9

Breaking the Silence

In April 2008 I was preparing to leave for Chicago to deliver a paper on condoms and AIDS prevention; I was still perplexed that the Vatican had taken so long to release the findings of its specially commissioned study on condoms/AIDS. Like everyone else, I was unaware of the Congregation for the Doctrine of Faith decision to shelve the report prepared by the office of Cardinal Barragán and to ignore requests for an update about it. I decided to make some phone calls. First on my list was Bishop Kevin Dowling; surely he would know the status of the report. I placed my very first call to Rustenburg, South Africa, and fortunately was able to get a clear answer to my question. The bishop did not know anything about the long-awaited report and so we were both in the dark. Everything at that time was very secretive and no one was sharing information, including some religion reporters. Austen Ivereigh was doing his sleuthing with trusted Vatican contacts, but unfortunately he was not writing about what he knew in 2008.

Finally in March 2009, Benedict XVI broke the Vatican's three years of silence and informed the public that there would be no change in Catholic Church teaching regarding condoms and AIDS. Nothing had changed since his June 2005 statement to African bishops. No special Vatican study was ever released, and no explanation was given for the non-delivery of the report promised in 2006. Ironically, he made this announcement to journalists during his first visit to Africa—a continent devastated by HIV/AIDS. While flying to Africa, he told reporters that the church's opposition to the use of condoms to prevent AIDS would remain in full effect: abstinence and fidelity were the best ways to avoid the disease.

He said that AIDS "cannot be overcome by the distribution of condoms. On the contrary, they increase the problem."[1] Here we see the "effectiveness" argument against condoms once again, which was first floated by Cardinal Trujillo in 2003. But Benedict raised the stakes even higher by the above comments. First, the Vatican told Catholics not to use condoms because that would be immoral and against church teaching; second, we were told that condoms did not work so do not use them; finally, in 2009, the pope said condoms should not be used because they "increase the problem."

This comment so enraged the health care community that the editors of Britain's prestigious medical journal *The Lancet* demanded a retraction, since the vast majority of scientific studies up to that point had demonstrated that the proper use of condoms reduced the likelihood of contracting sexually transmitted diseases, including HIV/AIDS.[2] *The Lancet* editors wrote: "Whether the Pope's error was due to ignorance or a deliberate attempt to manipulate science to support Catholic ideology is unclear. . . . When any influential person, be it a religious or political leader, makes a false scientific statement that could be devastating to the health of millions of people, they should retract or correct the public record. Anything less from Pope Benedict would be an immense disservice to the public and health advocates, including many thousands of Catholics who work tirelessly to try and prevent the spread of HIV/AIDS worldwide."[3] Neither the pope nor any Vatican official offered the retraction which medical experts had demanded. In the face of such international outrage, several groups—UNAIDS, the World Population Fund, and WHO—issued a joint statement saying that "the male latex condom is the single, most efficient, available technology to reduce the sexual transmission of HIV."[4]

In an attempt to bolster its stand against condoms to fight AIDS, the Vatican has repeatedly cited the work of Harvard anthropologist Edward Green,[5] who has stated in one context that condoms have not worked to stem the tide of HIV/AIDS infections in Africa's generalized epidemics. He argued that condoms alone will not solve the AIDS problem in Africa, but rather programs that foster, among other things, behavioral change (abstinence and fidelity) will make a difference. This is code for advocating partner reduction—a key variable in lowering the risk of contracting HIV/AIDS. Dr. Green has never asserted that condoms have no place in AIDS prevention, a point Catholic conservatives tend to ignore. He was invited to speak at a Vatican-sponsored AIDS conference in Rome, June 2011, but reform-minded clerics like Bishop Kevin Dowling were not.[6] Green's work and findings are formidable, but those who think he is opposed to condom use in Africa do not know the core principles of his work. The research findings that show condoms do not stop the spread of AIDS in Africa could be the result of inconsistent condom usage rather than the conclusion Rome wishes to draw: see we told you so, condoms do not work and cause more problems. Condom use in Africa had not reached a sufficiently high level to produce a measureable slowing of new infections. Green's final summary about the issue is unmistakable: "Don't misunderstand me; I am not anti-condom. All people should have full access to condoms, and condoms should always be a back-up strategy for those who will not or cannot remain in a mutually faithful relationship."[7] This is definitely not a Vatican mantra, and his statements, on balance, do not support Catholic teaching being expounded as of 2009.

It is clear from an extensive review of the literature that certain new and old interventions work to prevent the spread of HIV/AIDS.

1. For reasons not fully known at this time, research scientists have found that male circumcision reduces the risk of HIV infection in men. In African regions where male circumcision is almost universal, HIV prevalence is relatively low.[8] Since intercourse from a physiological point of view is a process of rubbing (penis and vagina), there are invariably instances wherein tears in the skin and tissue can occur—many at a microscopic level. This tearing/bleeding is less likely, on average, for the circumcised penis which exhibits what is called "keratinization" (toughening of skin) due to the surgical scar of circumcision. Hence, there is less likelihood of any blood flow and through it the passing on of the HIV to the male through this medium. The male benefits, not the female, but in the long run, with fewer infected males, women are better off. Malcolm Potts and associates state that unlike most other interventions, male circumcision is "a one-time procedure that confers lifelong protection." He continues that mathematical models suggest that male circumcision "could avert up to 5.7 million new HIV infections and 3 million deaths over the next twenty years in Sub-Saharan Africa, many of these among women."[9] Cindy Lui's research supports this conclusion, but for different reasons.[10] Her study demonstrates that circumcised males have less bacteria present immediately below the "head" of the penis and this helps block the route of HIV entry. Thus, Lui argues that circumcision lowers the risk of acquiring sexually transmitted viral infections, particularly HIV; the risk of contracting the virus falls to about 50–60 percent in the circumcised group.

   The next step is to determine the cost of large-scale programs to have males circumcised and convince locals that this procedure will save lives—maybe their own. The projected number of people who could benefit from circumcision programs must bring smiles to all health care workers. They can truly have a real impact on a deadly disease with the cooperation of medicine, science, government, and religion. Ten years ago we had no idea that circumcision had any relationship to the spread of HIV/AIDS. Aaron Tobian et al. summarize their research on circumcision this way: "These findings, in conjunction with those of previous trials, indicate that circumcision should now be accepted as an efficacious intervention for reducing heterosexually acquired infections with HSV-2, HPV, and HIV in adolescent boys and men. However, it must be emphasized that protection was only partial, and it is critical to promote the practice of safe sex."[11]

2. Since there is no single program that guarantees the prevention of AIDS, there are several factors which are important for HIV/AIDS education. Health care experts recommend behavioral change (abstinence, fidelity) as measured by reducing the number of sex partners and "consistent condom use." These factors, in combination, will provide some of the best results.

Because Vatican leaders have strongly opposed the use of condoms in any of their prevention programs, critics have labeled the Vatican an obstructionist in the worldwide quest for an effective AIDS prevention strategy. Later on, in a 2010 book-length interview with Peter Seewald, Pope Benedict complained that he was misunderstood by *The Lancet*, the media, and others: "In my remarks [March 17, 2009] I was not making a general statement about the condom issue, but merely said . . . that we cannot solve the problem by distributing condoms."[12] This appears to be a strange parsing of words since the key issue raised by papal critics since 2000 had always been the following: will the church allow Catholics to use condoms to prevent the spread of AIDS? Dr. Koop asked Americans to use condoms to prevent the spread of HIV/Aids in the 1980s. No responsible scholar has ever suggested that (1) simply distributing condoms in the town square would solve the AIDS problem; (2) nor were clerics within the pope's own denomination saying that pastors should distribute condoms to parishioners at church services. Nonetheless, many conservative Catholics defend the pope by saying he is opposed to the "distribution of condoms" as a cure-all. They seem to be implying that the pope had a point. No published medical scientist has ever subscribed to the idea that condoms are an absolute cure-all. Condoms are just one item in the medical tool box for the prevention of AIDS. It is an important one but not the proverbial "magic bullet." The real solution to the AIDS pandemic still eludes us, namely, "the development of an effective HIV vaccine. This challenge has been particularly difficult because of the nature of the virus, particularly its ability to integrate itself into the genome of host cells, to readily mutate, and to conceal that part of its outer coat that would induce protective antibodies."[13]

We are at a point in our discussion to answer some of the most persistent criticism of condom use. Why advocate the use of condoms, since they supposedly do not work and only make things worse?

- I simply respond to this by saying, why would bishops like Kevin Dowling and a host of others advocate the use of condoms to prevent the spread of AIDS if these ideas were not going to help their people? Are all the bishops who follow Dowling's lead incompetent? Hardly.
- In the 1980s and 1990s Dr. C. Everett Koop developed programs in the United States involving abstinence, fidelity, and safe sex (condom use). No one claimed that condoms were ineffective during this period of the AIDS epidemic since the rates of infection and death due to AIDS declined.
- Edward Green found that consistent use of condoms among sex workers in Thailand reduced the spread of AIDS in this high-risk group. He advocates the use of condoms in Africa together with programs that teach abstinence and fidelity.
- Finally, we consistently find peer-reviewed medical journals (e.g., Tobian et al., see above) advocating the practice of safe sex, condoms, and so on, no matter what the prevention program is. In Tobian's paper, male circumcision has proven to be effective in reducing the probability of getting AIDS, but these authors recommend practicing safe sex, too. Whether they are talking about male circumcision, antiretroviral drugs, or other issues, scientists frequently end up their speeches and articles by saying patients should practice safe sex. Would these authors or respected journals be articulating these ideas if "condoms increase the problem?" I don't think so.

The condom/AIDS debate continued in the Catholic Church in 2009 and part of 2010. Then a remarkable change occurred in Pope Benedict's thinking after five years of defending Pope John Paul's teaching—the first pope to ever talk about AIDS. In an interview with German writer Peter Seewald, Pope Benedict finally opened the door to the use of condoms to prevent AIDS. Some call this the "November surprise."

NOTES

1. Victor Simpson, "Pope Says Condoms Worsen HIV Problem," *Washington Post*, March 18, 2009.
2. See the appendix for a list of studies/authors that support the thesis that condoms help to prevent the spread of HIV/AIDS.

3. Editorial, "Redemption for the Pope?" *The Lancet* 373, no. 9669 (2009): 1054.
4. Editorial, "Redemption?" 1054.
5. Edward Green, *Rethinking AIDS Prevention: Learning from Successes in Developing Countries* (Westport, CT: Praeger, 2003); also read his book: *Broken Promises: How the AIDS Establishment Has Betrayed the Developing World* (Sausalito, CA: PoliPointPress, 2011).
6. www.huffingtonpost.com/2011/05/24/vatican-aids-condoms_n_866439.html (accessed June 23, 2013).
7. Edward Green, "The Pope May Be Right," *Washington Post*, March 29, 2009.
8. Malcolm Potts et al., "Reassessing HIV Prevention," *Science* 320, no. 5877 (2008): 750.
9. Potts, "Reassessing HIV," 750.
10. Cindy Liu et al., "Male Circumcision Significantly Reduces Prevalence and Load of Genital Anaerobic Bacteria," *mBio* 4, no. 2 (2013): e00076–13. DOI: 10.1128/mBio.00076-13.
11. Aaron Tobian et al., "Male Circumcision for the Prevention of HSV-2 and HPV Infections and Syphilis," *New England Journal of Medicine* 360 (March 26, 2009): 1302.
12. Benedict XVI, *Light of the World* (A Conversation with Peter Seewald), trans. Michael Miller and Adrian Walker (San Francisco: Ignatius Press, 2010), 118.
13. Anthony Fauci, "Twenty-Five Years of HIV/AIDS," March 25, 2007; www.project-syndicate.org/commentary/twenty-five-years-of-hiv-aids (accessed June 22, 2013).

10

Pope Benedict Sees the Light

We are now in a position to review the various ways Catholic Church leaders responded to the AIDS crisis. Cardinal Ratzinger objected to the U.S. bishops' statement on AIDS (1987) because it seemed to endorse immoral practices. A group of curial cardinals asserted that condoms were ineffective and so why use them. Finally, the pope stepped on the international scene and argued that the use of condoms only made things worse. With many high-level church officials objecting to Rome's stance on condoms and AIDS, no resolution of the conflict was in sight.

This book has taken the reader through the long and torturous journey from 1987 to the fifth year of Pope Benedict's pontificate, 2010. Table 10.1 gives the timeline of this religious struggle.[1]

It is clear that between 1981 and 1990 only three bishops/cardinals publicly registered their objections to Vatican policy on AIDS prevention. In the next ten years the number of dissidents almost tripled as the incidents of worldwide AIDS deaths surpassed 1.5 million per year. But between 2000 and 2010 fully twenty high-ranking clerics voiced their disapproval of Rome's directives on AIDS prevention. The two popes living during this period of controversy always stressed that the way to fight HIV/AIDS was through abstinence and fidelity, not by using condoms. Over three decades thirty-one dissidents came forward—including the U.S. Bishops' Administrative Board—to voice their objections to this papal doctrine and offered several explanations as to why the church should change its policy. Only a limited number of critics emerged before the year 2000. Then an avalanche of objections came rolling in, no doubt fueled by the realization that millions were dying of the dread disease,

Table 10.1. Timeline on Vatican dispute about using condoms to prevent AIDS.

Year	*Spokesperson(s)*	*Permit use of Condoms?*
1987	U.S. Bishops	Yes
1988	Cardinal Ratzinger	No
1988	Cardinal Lustiger	Yes
1989	Bishop Gaillot	Yes
1993	Archbishop Collini	Yes
1993	John Paul II	No
1996	Bishop Guazzelli	Yes
1996	Bishop Rouet	Yes
1996	Bishop Monteiro	Yes
1996	Cardinal Simonis	Yes
1996	Bishop Beuzeville	Yes
1996	Cardinal Schönborn	Yes
1999	Bishop Muskens	Yes
2000	Bishop Rixen	Yes
2001	Bishop Dowling (1)	Yes, change policy
2003	Archbishop Conti (1)	Yes
2003	Cardinal Trujillo	No
2004	Cardinal Danneels	Yes
2004	Cardinal Murphy-O'Connor	Yes
2005	Bishop Kamphaus	Yes
2005	Spain's Bishops	No*
2005	Belgian Bishops	Yes
2005	Bishop Arizmendi	Yes, change policy
2005	Archbishop Lele	Yes
2005	Cardinal Cottier	Yes, change policy
2005	Pope Benedict XVI	No
2005	Bishop Dowling (2)	Yes, change policy
2005	Cardinal Javier Barragán	Yes, change policy
2006	Cardinal Tumi	Yes
2006	Bishop Cote	Yes
2006	Bishop Moreira	Yes
2006	Archbishop Conti (2)	Yes
2006	Cardinal Martini	Yes, change policy
2006	Pope Benedict XVI	Timeout; call for a study
2009	Pope Benedict XVI	No
2009	Bishop Jaschke	Yes
2009	Bishop Clemente	Yes
2009	Bishop Ferreira	Yes
2010	Pope Benedict XVI	Yes, in some circumstances

*Some asked for a change in policy but that intervention failed.

but the Vatican would not budge. Some challengers argued that using a condom to prevent the spread of AIDS was the lesser of two evils. Others maintained that *Humanae Vitae* allowed exceptions to the ban on contraceptives for health reasons.

To the surprise of many Vatican observers, Pope Benedict presented a new twist on the Catholic/Condoms/AIDS debate in his book, *Light of the World* (2010). During six days of taped conversations (one hour each day) with journalist Peter Seewald in the summer of 2010, the pope was asked, among other things, about his stand on the use of condoms to fight HIV/AIDS. One would expect him to say that the best way to fight AIDS is through fidelity and abstinence. That is what he had been saying all along. Like John Paul II, one would expect Benedict to state that Catholics are not allowed to use condoms to prevent HIV/AIDS. Instead, after decades of papal pronouncements banning the use of condoms to prevent the spread of AIDS, Benedict had a change of heart. He said that in certain circumstances, it would be morally commendable to use a condom while having sex to prevent the spread of AIDS. Pope Benedict wrote: "There may be a basis in the case of some individuals, as perhaps when a male prostitute uses a condom, where this can be a first step in the direction of a moralization, a first assumption of responsibility."[2] The pope was clearly giving the public and Catholics in particular new information about how to deal with HIV/AIDS which he had not shared with them before. The hypothetical male prostitute was being morally responsible up to a point, Benedict said. The man had made the first step. Later on, Peter Seewald followed with the question: "Are you saying, then, that the Catholic Church is actually not opposed in principle to the use of condoms?" The Pope answered: "She of course does not regard it as a real or moral solution, but, in this or that case, there can be nonetheless, in the intention of reducing the risk of infection, a first step in a movement toward a different way, a more human way, of living sexuality."[3] Yes, he said such behavior was a more human way of doing things.

No one can doubt that the pope was suggesting that Catholics take the first step to a higher moral life. And certainly he would want Catholics to move in this more human way. It is important to note here that there is no reference to his previous statement that condoms "increase the problem." One cannot commend a person for reducing the risk of infection by using a condom and at the same time assert that such action will "increase the problem." The pope at this point in 2010 had apparently dropped that idea completely. But lest anyone think that Pope Benedict was caught off guard by an unfriendly journalist's question, Seewald states the following in the book's preface: "In authorizing the text, the pope did not change the spoken word, and made only small corrections where he considered greater factual precision necessary."[4] In short, one must conclude that the words of Benedict were carefully crafted so as to present his true ideas as of November 2010, when the book was released to the public.

A barrage of media comments followed the publication of key parts of the pope's new book in the Vatican's official newspaper *L'Osservatore Romano* (Nov. 20, 2010) and elsewhere. James Martin, SJ, of *America* magazine offered these initial observations. He said that the pope's remarks were certainly a departure from previous teaching, an exception where there had never been an exception before. "While some bishops and archbishops have spoken in this way, the pope has never affirmed this," Martin said. "And it's interesting that he uses as an example someone who is trying to act morally to someone else by not passing on an infection, which was always the stance of those people who favored condoms in cases of HIV and AIDS. So it does mark a departure."[5]

Georgetown University scholar Fr. Thomas Reese, SJ, took a similar view, but points out that these papal comments certainly mean that the Catholic Church no longer espouses the view that condoms are intrinsically evil; he says the "pope's new statement blasts that idea out of the water."[6] He is obviously aware of fellow Jesuit cardinal Avery Dulles's observation that John Paul II was the only pope to ever say condoms are intrinsically evil. For a long time the word Catholics heard from the Vatican was that artificial birth control was intrinsically evil, and therefore, condoms were evil. Pope Benedict moved away from that position in 2010 and joined Pope Paul's birth control commission, which voted to scrap that idea in the 1960s. Slow and plodding has always been a hallmark of Pope Benedict. Fr. Federico Lombardi, director of the Vatican press office, subsequently clarified the pope's remarks and stated that Benedict's intention was not to distinguish between male or female prostitutes. Rather, Lombardi said: "If it is a man, a woman or a transsexual who does it [uses a condom], we are always at the same point, which is the first step in responsibly avoiding passing on a grave risk to the other."[7] So these remarks and clarifications point in one direction: the prostitute is doing a morally good thing by using a condom. No question about that. In the words of certain social theorists, we are now observing a period of "settlement" in the Catholic Church where opposing fields assess their positions and make changes. This can be a long and drawn out process.[8] Our study shows that it takes considerable time for church leaders to embrace the proper health care program and join medical science in resolving key problems. That is one of the sad realities of this investigation: the longer it takes to solve certain problems, the more lives are lost.

Of course, there were some Catholics who did not appreciate the pope's new stance on condoms and AIDS, even though numerous bishops and cardinals throughout the world had previously asked him to change his views to save lives. John Haas, who writes for *Our Sunday Visitor* and the conservative *Legatus Magazine*, had this unbelievable reaction to the pope's new book, *Light of the World*: "I told the publisher, 'Don't publish this; it's going to create such a mess.'"[9] These are strange words from a conservative Catholic who advocates loyalty and obedience to the successor of St. Peter as a core belief. And, who ever heard of someone telling a publisher not to print a colleague's book—especially one written by a pope? That is like having a grad student condemning a book written by the president of Harvard.

Some priests from the Catholic right were dismayed as well. "I'm sorry. I love the Holy Father very much; he is a deeply holy man and has done a great deal for the church," Father Tim Finigan, a British priest wrote, but "on this particular issue, I disagree with him."[10] After years of Catholic controversies, these are the reactions we expect to hear from liberals like Küng, Martini, and Curran, but from conservative Fr. Finigan? He has fallen into the trap set for all progressives: Got Ya! You're a cafeteria Catholic! It signifies a Catholic who takes one teaching or practice but skips over another he or she does not like. It is amazing what people will do when caught off guard—when they assert their fundamentalist views and not the traditional Catholic mantra which for conservatives is: the pope is the Vicar of Christ; he has got to be right. We should obey him.

Obviously, major differences still exist in the Catholic Church on this topic which has festered for some twenty-five years. Nevertheless, the pope has made it obvious that his thinking has changed from his speech to African bishops in June 2005, when he told them that the "spread of HIV and AIDS in Africa should be tackled through fidelity and abstinence and not by condoms."[11] With about thirty-four-million people living with HIV/AIDS worldwide, it became clear that widely accepted prevention techniques had to become a priority of the Catholic Church.

The papal shock wave caught conservative Catholic scholar George Weigel by surprise; he thought it was imprudent for the pope to have this discussion in a journalistic interview. One wonders what he thought of Pius XII's decision to give a special address about birth control to Italian midwives and related professionals (1951). Ironically, Weigel wrote the forward to the pope's new book, *Light of the World*, and never mentioned his reservations about Benedict's views in that essay. Rather he heaped praise on the book by saying Peter Seewald's "well-crafted questions give Benedict XVI good material with which to work. But it is the remarkably lucid and precise mind of Joseph Ratzinger that makes the papal answers here sing."[12] One wonders if the man actually read the book before it was published. Moreover, this is an odd turn of events in the so-called consistent mind of a conservative theologian. But maybe not. Weigel made a serious error by overstating the findings of the Edward Green study[13] on condoms and AIDS in 2009. Green's research demonstrates that among high-risk groups such as prostitutes in Thailand and Cambodia, condom use has a marked effect in reducing the transmission of HIV.[14] For some reason, probably because of low rates of condom usage and ethnic tribal norms, the same results have not been found thus far in Africa. Consistent condom use in the United States, Asia, and Europe has helped reduce the spread of AIDs in those countries, according to the CDC.[15] Weigel failed to note that Green maintains that condoms "should have a back-up role even in the generalized epidemics of Africa. I believe condoms should be made available to everyone. It should be, and as you say, the ABC strategy: *A*bstain, *B*e faithful, use a Condom [emphasis mine]."[16] Cafeteria Catholics breed cafeteria research.

I find it amazing that conservative Catholics agree with the Holy Father (Paul VI) who wrote *Humanae Vitae,* which condemned birth control and condoms as did the writings of John Paul II, but then they go and beg to differ with the Holy Father (Benedict) who applies previously articulated Catholic principles to new situations and problems: the crisis of AIDS. Ideology is mightier than the catechism. Thirty days after the "November Surprise," Rome's Congregation for the Doctrine of the Faith (CDF) issued a formal statement clarifying the pope's remarks in his new book, *Light of the World.*[17] Thus we have a statement from an official Vatican source and do not have to rely on an interview published in a new book one can buy at Barnes and Noble. First, CDF stated that the pope's new book is not breaking with the church's doctrine concerning contraception as outlined in *Humanae Vitae.* That was never an issue. Second, the CDF wanted to inform Catholics that, in the pope's view, condoms do not constitute a "real or moral solution" to the problem of AIDS. Of course, when dealing with a disease like HIV/AIDS, one has to admit that the "real" solution is to find a vaccine to protect children, mothers, and all humanity from sickness and possible death. The ethical imperative, the moral mandate, is "Thou shalt not Kill" (Deut. 5:17), and so cardinals and bishops around the world had asked the Vatican to permit the use of condoms to help prevent AIDS. Catholics must not put others at risk for getting a possible deadly disease. That was the moral issue at stake. The pope praises the higher morality of the prostitute who, when using a condom, is moving toward a more human way of living. Furthermore, the document from CDF emphasizes in a third point that "it cannot be denied that anyone who uses a condom in order to diminish the risk posed to another person is intending to reduce the evil connected with his or her immoral activity. In this sense the Holy Father points out that the use of a condom 'with the intention of reducing the risk of infection, can be a first step in a movement towards a different way, a more human way, of living sexuality.'" In short, the CDF is affirming that "those involved in prostitution who are HIV positive and who seek to diminish the risk of contagion by the use of a condom may be taking the first step in respecting the life of another." It should be noted that the prefect of CDF at this time, Cardinal William Levada, uses the term "prostitute" without regard to the person's gender. Lastly, the CDF text notes that the "Church teaches that prostitution is immoral and should be shunned."[18] This hardly needs mentioning. In conclusion, the CDF is stating, with the pope, that in certain circumstances, the utilization of condoms to prevent HIV/AIDS can be a positive first step in respecting life and preventing AIDS. We might add that anyone whose actions reduce evil is to be commended, according to Benedict.

As noted previously, many authors have decided to comment on this papal U-turn of sorts. One of the most insightful essays on Benedict's new book, *Light of the World,* is one written by Fr. Anthony Egan, SJ. He states that Benedict provides some subtle innovations on the use of condoms to prevent the spread of AIDS and makes three crucial observations in his essay. First, he says many Catholics have forgotten that *Humanae Vitae* contains a special medical exemption that is not well known in Catholic theological circles. Pope Paul VI maintained that "the Church does not consider at all illicit the use of those therapeutic means necessary to cure bodily diseases, even if a foreseeable impediment to procreation should result there from—provided such impediment is not directly intended for any motive whatsoever."[19] Second, Egan thinks that Benedict's insights and change in direction are an application of the *Humanae Vitae* exemption clause, namely, an action is not illicit if it is not intended. Such an observation leads to the conclusion that using a condom during intercourse has a "bad effect" because there is no chance for conception, but that is a side effect of the intended good effect (prevention of HIV infection). A third and final point made by Egan is that "the Pope is in fact implicitly applying this clause of *Humanae Vitae* to the present situation."[20] What the pope has asserted in *Light of the World* is in reality the basic thesis of Martin Rhonheimer's article published in 2004 and discussed above in chapter 5 of this book. The article makes two points which we ought to review.

First, Rhonheimer asserted that not every sexual act in which a condom is used is contraceptive (two men having sex). Using a condom in this instance has one meaning and one meaning alone and that is prevention. The person who has HIV hopefully does not want to infect his or her partner. Second, the CDF consultant turns to the issue of married couples. He argues that "a married man who is HIV-infected and uses a condom to protect his wife from infection is not acting to render procreation impossible, but to prevent infection. If conception is prevented, this will be an 'unintentional' side-effect and will not therefore shape the moral meaning of the act as a contraceptive act."[21] We are now in a position to say that

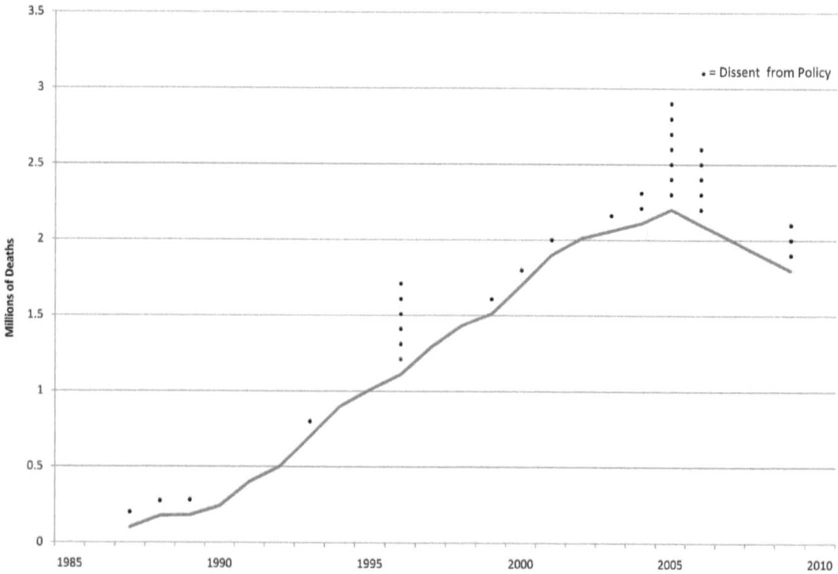

Figure 10.1. Deaths Worldwide due to AIDS by Year (in millions) and Cleric Dissidents. UNAIDS, Report on the Global AIDS Epidemic, 2010.

whether one is talking about two men having sex or a married couple, the use of a condom to prevent the spread of AIDS is the correct thing to do. The statements of Pope Benedict, who was once head of the CDF while Rhonheimer worked there as a consultant show a remarkable coalescence in their thinking. The seeds for change were planted in 2004 by Rhoheimer, but the pope only came around to this line of thinking in 2010. In addition, the data presented in figure 10.1 show that the two popes were under tremendous pressure from episcopal colleagues to make a change in church policy. Almost twenty bishops and cardinals registered their objections to papal policy after 2004. The engine that drove such responses was the mounting casualties due to AIDS.

Benedict has shown over time a shift in thinking and a willingness to embrace the ideas of contemporary moral theologians and some bishops. What we have uncovered is a medical ethics issue embedded in a sexual morality question. The health of the individual comes first. The conclusion is that he realized that saving lives trumps all issues related to the condoms-AIDS debate.

In a sense, Ratzinger is the beginning and end of the AIDS/Condom debate for Catholics. In 1987 he chided the U.S. bishops for developing AIDS prevention programs which included instructions on using condoms to prevent HIV. Later on, his views changed a bit so that he could say in 2010 that under certain conditions one could use a condom to avoid passing on the AIDS disease to one's partner. It is a crucial move forward—a modest statement of progress after about twenty-five years of theological wrangling.

In conclusion, the CDF document clarifies and makes official what the pope said during interviews with Peter Seewald, namely, that in some circumstances the use of condoms to prevent a deadly disease is morally commendable because it reduces the possible harm to other human beings by not exposing them to the risk of HIV/AIDS. That is not a trivial matter; it is a move forward for the individual and the church. Ivereigh comments on the new teaching of Benedict this way:

> The breakthrough is the Pope's mention of a condom as a positive first step—impossible were it "intrinsically evil." It is a rejection of the misuse of church teaching by self-appointed guardians of orthodoxy. There is no doubt what he meant, and he has articulated the mind of the Church. Agencies on the front line can breathe more easily now.[22]

NOTES

1. These names were collected by determining which bishop(s) first objected to Vatican policy on HIV/AIDS utilizing the *New York Times.* Second, I checked the *National Catholic Reporter* for its list of dissenters. Third, I consulted Catholics for Choice, Washington, D.C.
2. Benedict XVI, *Light of the World* (A Conversation with Peter Seewald) (San Francisco: Ignatius Press, 2010), 119.
3. Benedict XVI, *Light,* 119–20.
4. Benedict XVI, *Light,* xix.
5. James Martin comments: www.nbcnews.com/id/40289256/ns/world_news-europe/#.Ucm_ZpzeYpo (accessed June 15, 2013).
6. Thomas Reese, "Sex and the Fifth Commandment," *Washington Post,* November 22, 2010.
7. Philip Pullella, "Vatican Broadens Case for Condoms to Fight AIDS," Reuters, November 24, 2010; http://blogs.reuters.com/faithworld/2010/11/24/vatican-broadens-case-for-condoms-to-fight-aids/ (accessed June 23, 2013).
8. Neil Fligstein and Doug McAdam, "Toward a General Theory of Strategic Action Fields," *Sociological Theory* 29 (2011): 2, 18.
9. Quoted in Rachel Donadio and Laurie Goodstein, "After Condom Remarks, Vatican Confirms Shift," *New York Times,* November 23, 2010.
10. Quoted in David Gibson, "The Catholic Church, Condoms and 'Lesser Evils,'" *New York Times,* November 27, 2010.
11. *BBC News,* "Pope Rejects Condoms for Africa," http://news.bbc.co.uk/2/hi/4081276.stm (accessed May 15, 2012).
12. Benedict XVI, *Light,* xi–xii.
13. Edward Green, *Rethinking AIDS Prevention* (Westport, CT: Praeger, 2003).

14. William Crawley, "The Pope Was Right about Condoms, Says Harvard HIV expert," BBC News, March 29, 2009; www.bbc.co.uk/blogs/ni/2009/03/aids_expert_who_defended_the_p.html (accessed June 19, 2012).

15. CDC, "Condoms and STDs," September 13, 2011; www.cdc.gov/condomeffectiveness/latex.htm (accessed June 1, 2012).

16. Edward Green Comments: www.bbc.co.uk/blogs/ni/2009/03/aids_expert_who_defended_the_p.html; (accessed March 18, 2011).

17. Congregation for the Doctrine of the Faith (CDF), "Note on the Banalization of Sexuality Regarding Certain Interpretations of 'Light of the World,'" Rome, December 21, 2010.

18. CDF, "Note on the Banalization."

19. Paul VI, *Humanae Vitae* (Boston, MA: St. Paul books and media, 1968) par. 15.

20. Anthony Egan, "The Pope on Condoms: Change or No Change?" *Thinking Faith: The Online Journal of the British Jesuits*, November 24, 2010; www.thinkingfaith.org/articles/20101124_2.htm (accessed April 17, 2012).

21. Martin Rhonheimer, "The Truth about Condoms," *The Tablet*, July 10, 2004.

22. Austin Ivereigh, "Towards a New Morality: Condoms and Church Teaching," *The Tablet*, November 27, 2010, 1–2.

11

+

Counting the Cost

The Vatican breakthrough amounted to rethinking the medical ethics principles that were well-known but had not yet been applied to this new disease. The secular world had its own reaction to Benedict's statement: "It's about time," snapped a physician who was being interviewed during a morning TV news program after the November surprise. The Catholic Church's decision makers demonstrated that they move at a snail's pace even when lives are at stake. As we come to the end of our journey about condoms, AIDS, and the Catholic Church, this simple question comes to mind: What if church officials would have acted sooner? What if John Paul II had listened to Cardinal Lustiger in 1988? What if Benedict XVI had acted immediately upon the advice of Cardinal Martini in 2006? Obviously, things would have turned out differently for thousands of people . . . but how many?

The "What if?" is a well-known tool used by social historians to make a point. I do not consider this line of questioning an exercise for amateurs who cannot figure out what to do with their spare time. Many eminent historians have looked back at important events in our social world and speculated about what would have happened if just the opposite action occurred in history. Here are some examples:

- What if John F. Kennedy was never assassinated?
- Two-time Pulitzer Prize–winning historian Robert McCullough has pondered, "What if George Washington's retreat after the battle of Long Island had not succeeded?"

- John Stacks and Lawrence Malkin ask, "What if Watergate were still just an upscale address?"
- What if the Mayflower had never set sail?

Following this well-known literary device, I have decided to ask this question: What if the previous two popes (John Paul II and Benedict XVI) had never banned the use of condoms to prevent the spread of AIDS? What if pastors were told to encourage people from the pulpit and in the Sunday bulletin to be sure to use a condom if they were HIV positive because it was the right thing to do? How would this have changed the course of history and saved lives?

We know this could have happened because of the following three historical facts. First, it is obvious that many bishops and cardinals advocated the use of condoms to prevent the spread of AIDS, starting as early as the mid-1980s. They were leaders in the church and felt strongly that it was the moral thing to do, despite papal pronouncements to the contrary. Second, writers such as Marcella Alsan, MD, Peter Piot, and Nicholas Kristof have lamented that thousands—maybe millions—of lives have been lost because of the Catholic policy on condoms and AIDS. These are powerful assertions which irk many conservative Catholics who think the Vatican was right in banning condoms. Third, social and behavioral scientists such as Edward Green of Harvard and others have advocated a program of A + B + C for both poor and rich countries. That program of behavior change (abstinence and fidelity) together with condoms as a back-up plan provides one of the best chances to reduce the spread of AIDS. We have read the opinions of these experts for many years. So, we ask again: what if the Catholic Church early on would have approved a program to use condoms to fight the spread of AIDS? The three above groups would probably say "YES, they should have done this a long time ago." Do we have any idea about the impact of such a hypothetical program if it had been implemented? Not precisely, but we can try to give a reasonable and thoughtful answer to the question.

The cumulative number of deaths worldwide as the result of AIDS was estimated to be 24 million in 2007 by John Bongaarts et al. of the Population Council. Scholars are aware that this number is probably an undercount, given the discoveries of Peter Piot and others. He has recently tested old blood vials from Africa (1976) and found HIV present in them. The Bongaarts group uses the best methodology to gather global AIDS statistics, and so we will utilize their database for this discussion despite its limitations. By 2009 the number of AIDS-related deaths stood at 27.8 million based on my own calculations using UNAIDS data for years 2008 and 2009 (figure 11.1).

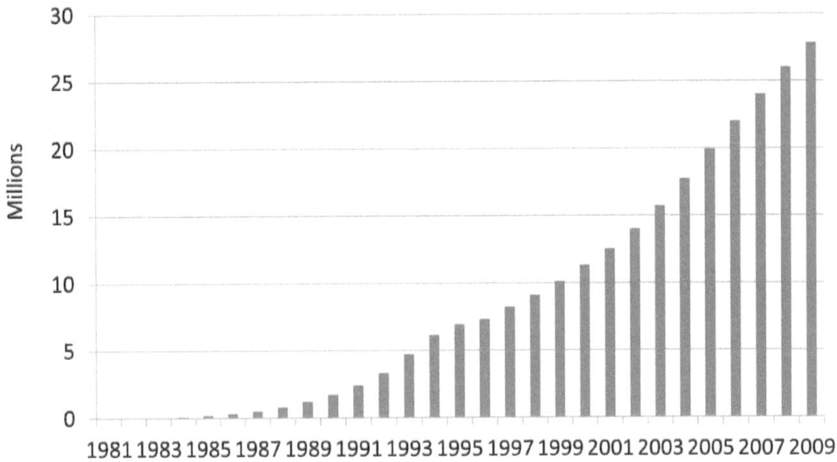

Figure 11.1. Cumulative AIDS Deaths Worldwide, 1981–2009. UNAIDS, Global Report, 2010.

These grim statistics tell us what has happened to the human race since 1981 when we began collecting reliable AIDS data. This disease is no ordinary pandemic; it is a "lethal illness with far-reaching implications for individuals, families, communities, health care providers and delivery systems. . . . It has become the leading infectious cause of mortality worldwide."[1] For about three decades health care workers and scientists have been fighting this disease, and they have been able to limit its deadly effects to 27.8 million by the end of 2009. The total number of casualties could have been much worse without the heroic efforts on the part of many health care workers. We can only speculate about how much higher these numbers would have been without the concerted efforts of thousands of health care professionals and the generous grants from major research foundations throughout the world. About 14 percent of the deaths represented in figure 11.1 are children (ages zero to fourteen).[2]

We now turn to the central question of this chapter, "What if?"—what if the Catholic Church had developed a viable program based on high quality medical and scientific research to deal with AIDS prevention during the period when many bishops were asking for change? Figure 11.2 below offers some reasonable estimates that we might have expected from a program initiated by Catholic Church officials in 2002, if they had listened to the many bishops and cardinals who had called for reform.

With three years of preparation, testing, and communication regarding the program, we have assembled some real and hypothetical data on preventable AIDS deaths that one could expect to find beginning in 2005. The columns in gray are *actual* worldwide deaths due to AIDS that come

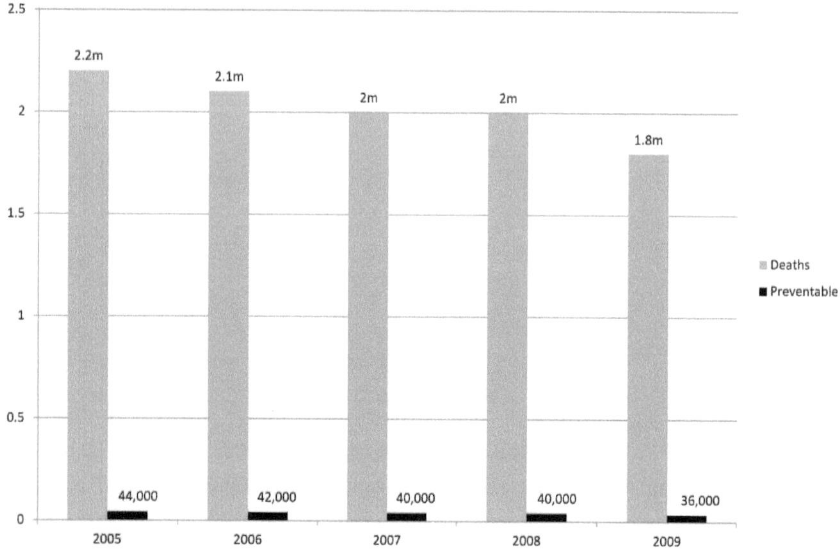

Figure 11.2. Actual Deaths (in millions) vs. Preventable Deaths (in thousands). UNAIDS, Global Report, 2010.

primarily from the calculations of Bongaarts and associates.[3] This study takes a rather conservative view regarding program outcomes and posits that we could possibly observe a 2 percent reduction (black columns) in AIDS deaths each year (2005–2009) throughout the world due to the new Catholic program, namely, an agreement to encourage the use of condoms to prevent AIDS. This intervention model assumes that the Catholic Church aggressively promotes a program that allows its members to use condoms to prevent the spread of AIDS and save lives. The above hypothesis is not unreasonable given the fact that there are approximately 1.2 billion Catholics (16.9 percent of world's population)[4] on the planet today, and the church has four-hundred-thousand priests on the payroll who could deliver the papal message. Using all aspects of media communication, the target population would be all Catholics in the world. We have not even mentioned the involvement of lay ministers (male and female) who certainly would be a major part of the program. The idea that such a program would achieve the modest effect outlined in figure 11.3 is definitely within the realm of possibility. The Centers for Disease Control states, "*Overall, the preponderance of available epidemiologic studies have found that when used consistently and correctly, condoms are highly effective in preventing the sexual transmission of HIV infection and reduce the risk of other STDs.*"[5] The goal is to reduce the number of HIV infections and deaths caused by AIDS and here are the figures we would expect in the five-year Catholic program. In 2005, instead of 2.2 million deaths, the 2 percent reduction due to the new program approved by Catholic leaders would cut the number of AIDS casualties in that year by 44,000 (in black). With 2.1 million deaths expected in 2006, we would reduce that number by 42,000 because of the 2 percent effect, and so on. In figure 11.2 one can see the projected reduction in years 2007, 2008, and 2009. Of course other factors will be at work to lessen the number of deaths worldwide due to AIDS. Health care experts hope to have more antiretroviral drugs available in years to come which will further cut the number of deaths to some degree. Unfortunately only about half of those who need antiretroviral drugs today actually receive them.[6] The poorest countries have the least access to these life-saving treatments. With fewer people getting infected by the HIV virus (use of condoms becomes a priority for more people), the overall number of AIDS deaths would drop considerably. Fewer people would need antiretroviral drugs (they have not become HIV infected) and that would save scarce health care dollars. In the five years we have selected for our study, we estimate that the total number of lives saved through the Catholic prevention model would have been 202,000 (44,000 + 42,000 + 40,000 + 40,000 + 36,000 = 202,000). Nicholas Kristof of the *New York Times* has said that the "Vatican's ban on condoms has cost many hundreds of thousands of lives from AIDS." We agree and feel his numbers are plausible. Marcella Alsan goes even further and says that the church's opposition to the use of condoms may have meant the loss of millions of lives. The numbers these people in the field are proposing leave the ordinary reader breathless.

The proposed Catholic prevention model not only would reduce death rates, but it could change the trajectory of HIV infections for years to come. In figure 11.3 we present some real and hypothetical data on HIV infections had the Catholic model been implemented fully in 2005.

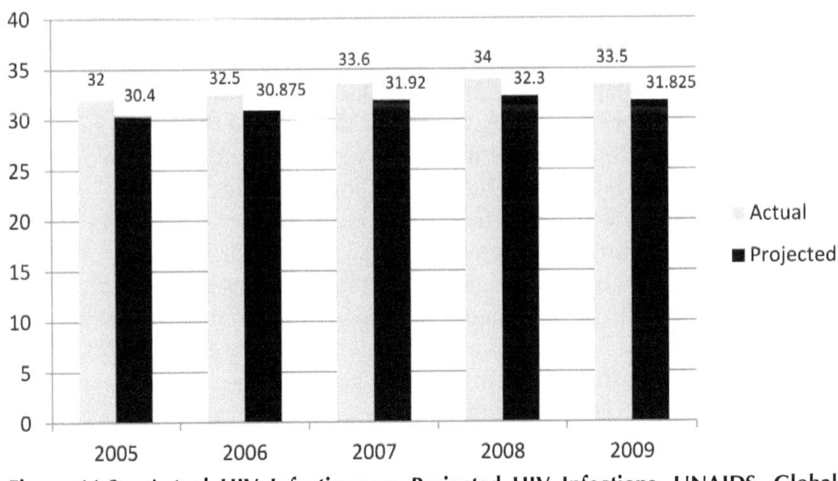

Figure 11.3. Actual HIV Infections vs. Projected HIV Infections. UNAIDS, Global Report, 2010.

Table 11.1. Summary of the projected reduction of HIV infections (millions) worldwide: 2005–2009.

Year	*Actual HIV Infections*	*Projected HIV Infections*	*Number Reduced*
2005	32	30.4	1.6
2006	32.5	30.875	1.63
2007	33.6	31.92	1.68
2008	34	32.3	1.7
2009	33.5	31.825	1.66
			Total: 8.27 million

In this discussion we project a modest 5-percent reduction in HIV infections as the result of the new Catholic initiative. In the year 2005 the total number of people living with HIV/AIDS was about 32 million, but if the Catholic program would have been implemented by then, we estimate that the number infected worldwide would have been reduced to 30.4 million—roughly a million and a half reduction. A modest 5-percent reduction could have meant a significant number of lives saved and a major reduction in the use of expensive antiretroviral drugs. In 2006 the new program would have resulted in about 1.6 million fewer HIV infections because condoms had become a significant part of the Catholic program to fight AIDS. Table 11.1 summarizes the overall program benefits over five years.

The cumulative effect of the Catholic program, if implemented, would have resulted in approximately eight million fewer HIV infections worldwide during the five-year period under consideration.

What this study has done for readers is provide a conservative estimate as to what the Catholic model could do for its members and many others who do not belong to the church, but who rely on Catholic-sponsored clinics for health care. It is well known that Catholic hospitals and clinics serve Catholics and non-Catholics alike, and so there is a chance for a greater impact with this program when we include the broad range of patients these health care facilities actually serve. The program would no doubt touch the lives of more than 1.2 billion Catholics.

Of course, some have said that AIDS is no longer a hot topic and is gradually fading into the woodwork as an important health issue. John Bongaarts and his colleagues[7] are not buying that argument at all. They point out that if all factors related to this disease remain constant, the cumulative death toll for AIDS in 2030 will be seventy-five million. Thus, it is not too late for implementing change, despite the church's many failures to act upon the recommendations of bishops throughout the world. There are millions of lives to be saved if effective programs become a part of all social and religious service agencies.

Many at the Vatican ought to apologize for past failings and admit their mistakes. Thomas Reese, SJ, thinks there are some bishops who should "lay down their crosiers" because they failed to properly manage the priest sexual-abuse problem in the Catholic Church.[8] It would not be out of place for those church leaders who handled the AIDS crisis so poorly to do the same; many lives have been lost and this calls for serious church reform and accountability. No one I know, however, is counting on that to happen very soon. The words of Dr. Alsan bear repeating; the church's opposition to the use of condoms "may mean not only untold human suffering, but the loss of millions of human lives." It is time to turn the page on the past and promise Catholics that church officials have learned their lesson and there will be no repeat fiascos in the future.

NOTES

1. William Cockerham, *Medical Sociology*, 12th ed. (New York: Prentice Hall, 2012), 37
2. John Bongaarts, Francois Pelletier, and Patrick Gerland, "Global Trends in AIDS Mortality," Working Paper #16, Population Council, New York, 2009: 7.
3. John Bongaarts, Francois Pelletier, and Patrick Gerland, "How Many More AIDS Deaths?" *Lancet* 375 (2010): 103.
4. U.S. Census Bureau, Population Clock, estimates the world population to be 7,094,310,470, June 26, 2013.
5. CDC, "Condom Effectiveness"; www.cdc.gov/condomeffectiveness/latex.htm (accessed April 14, 2013).
6. Erin Loury, "Scientists Make Curing HIV a Priority," *Los Angeles Times*, July 23, 2012.
7. John Bongaarts, "Global Trends," 6–7.
8. Thomas Reese, "On Sex Abuse," *America*, May 10, 2012.

12

+

Conclusion

The end of a book is like the end of a college course. We should ask ourselves, "What have we learned?" Simply put, one would have to conclude after reading the previous chapters that a great church faced a gigantic social problem and once again showed its flawed approach to dealing with the perplexities of modern life. These flaws became the "last lecture" of Cardinal Martini before he died, when he lamented that "the Church is two hundred years behind the times," and therefore he "called for it to recognize its mistakes and embark on a radical journey of change."[1] This is a shocking indictment of the post–Vatican II church by one of its principal leaders in the last forty years; it is a call for reform amidst organizational chaos.

PROBLEM: POPES RULE

We know that the Catholic Church has failed its families and many children when it mismanaged the sexual abuse crisis caused by priests and bishops in the previous five decades. Many are convinced that the church failed its members years ago by not allowing priests the option to marry. Numerous churches are without a pastor in Europe, and church closings due to a chronic priest shortage are a regular occurrence in the United States. Every day the church faces the fact that its policies deny women equal opportunities in its all-male clerical structure: they cannot be ordained to the priesthood. But in each of these failures no one has died as a result of church hyper-conservative policies.

The subject matter of this book, in contrast, opens a whole new chapter in the history of religious research. Nowhere today do we find major religious denominations taking a stand that would put its members at risk for getting a life-threatening disease, except for one. The Roman Catholic Church put its 1.2 billion members at risk for over thirty years. Only reluctantly did a pope in 2010 acknowledge that if Catholics have HIV/AIDS, they would be permitted to use a condom to prevent the spread of a deadly disease. By failing to allow its members the use of condoms to prevent the spread of AIDS early on, the top leadership of the church contributed to the deaths of thousands—perhaps millions. This is not my opinion alone, but that of numerous scholars inside and outside the church. What kind of distorted thinking causes religious people to act this way? It all began over one hundred years ago.

1. In 1870, during the proceedings of Vatican I, Pius IX felt it was necessary to assert explicitly a crucial prerogative of the Petrine office, that is, the doctrine of papal infallibility. The council agreed. When popes speak from the chair of Peter (ex cathedra) on faith and morals, according to Vatican I and subsequent clarifications, they cannot be wrong, otherwise they could lead the flock astray and jeopardize members' eternal salvation. The 1850s and 1860s had seen a resurgence of anti-Catholicism in Germany and other parts of Europe. Otto von Bismarck led the way with verbal attacks on religious orders, priests, and the pope himself. Perhaps Pius IX felt it was necessary at that time to remind the world of his supreme power and authority. This action led to an exaggeration of papal power and teaching authority during the next one hundred years; it would be corrected by Vatican II's insistence on the principle of collegiality such that popes and bishops by council decree work together to become pastors and not dictators.
2. The aftermath of Vatican I saw subsequent popes use this doctrine to declare, without reservation, certain dogmas of the faith, for example, that the Blessed Mother was assumed body and soul into heaven (Pius XII, 1950). Her corpse is not here on earth. Such a declaration has no biblical foundation whatsoever, but that did not seem to bother the pope and other church officials from declaring another Marian dogma. When Pius XI (1930) stated categorically that artificial birth control was immoral and forbidden to all Catholic married couples, however, it was unclear to many whether this was an infallible pronouncement and hence irreformable or simply a good sermon condemning the sin du jour. Be that as it may, subsequent popes *treated* this pronouncement as core Catholic teaching and not to be altered. Pius XII, Paul VI, John Paul II, and Benedict XVI never

seemed to waver in their support of Pius XI's teaching spelled out in the encyclical *Casti Connubii.* John XXIII, in contrast, saw that, during the Second Vatican Council, there were legitimate questions being raised regarding the artificial birth control issue, and so he appointed a special commission to study the matter. He was the only pope in recent times that had the temerity to ask the simple question: is this the Catholic Church's final statement on birth control? Paul VI slavishly followed the doctrine of Pius XI despite the birth control commission's recommendations to the contrary, and thus no change emerged on this front. Ottaviani got his way (semper idem, always the same). As time passed, the "no birth control" teaching became standard fare for all seminary moral theology courses from 1970 to 2010. It was seen as orthodox doctrine especially after the promulgation of Pope Paul VI's 1968 encyclical *Humanae Vitae,* even though several underhanded tactics were used to promote this teaching. The popes had spoken. So when 1981 rolled around and AIDS was declared a major health problem, Catholics had a limited set of options on how to respond.

3. AIDS and the pope: When John Paul II became the first pope to deal with the AIDS controversy, the shadow of previous anti–birth control administrations hung over the Vatican like a giant shroud. Since this pope helped write the document *Humanae Vitae,* according to some reports,[2] there was little doubt where he stood: there would be no birth control for Catholics, and condoms were evil. Thus, the Vatican made it clear to all Catholics that they should not use condoms to fight AIDS; that would be against long-standing Catholic tradition. Rather, they should either abstain from sex or be faithful to one's spouse. John Paul II and Benedict XVI hitched their theological wagon to a long tradition of anti–birth control Catholic teaching. They were frozen in time by past pronouncements and their own socialization process; they could not move beyond the thinking of their predecessors.

After all, we are not talking here about theologians, priests, or bishops. These are popes who are making major theological claims. It was much harder to change a crucial papal pronouncement after Vatican I than before. In the 1980s, papal paralysis was first observed in John Paul II. He stiffened his neck and back; he then bellowed out many times during his papacy that there would be no compromise even if lives were at stake. That was the substance of his teaching. Because papal policy automatically connected the use of condoms to prevent AIDS with previous papal pronouncements condemning contraceptives as gravely immoral, there was no chance for change or discussion. Previous papal teaching was assumed to be God's will.

PATH TO CHURCH FAILURE

This final review shows how powerful core beliefs dominated institutional Catholic Church culture in the previous one hundred years, especially ones articulated by former popes about immoral sexual practices. A sitting pope does not take lightly the dictates of his predecessors. Past papal teachings can make intelligent men fly in the face of facts, reason, and pastoral advice from respected colleagues. Very few active bishops in recent years would even allow a discussion regarding a major theological matter if a pope issued a decree against it. A summary of what has happened during the time period of this case study is outlined in four parts.

In the period of Catholic *reform,* John XXIII tried and succeeded to some degree in bringing change to a stagnant, post-war Catholic Church. For the most part the council supported his signature call of *aggiornamento.* What followed was a period of *dissent* by Catholic progressives and conservatives; until about 1980 these ecclesiastical rumblings were tolerated for the most part. Then a third phase of church organizational behavior was ushered in and was rightly called *restoration.* John Paul II, Cardinal Ratzinger, and others tried to halt the wave of change brought about by Vatican II and were somewhat successful. Collegiality was a dirty word, and those who did not conform to papal teaching were punished. By about the year 2000, forces in the church began to react to ecclesiastical scandals, errors, and outright sinfulness. We are now in a period of *accountability,* which could lead to meaningful reform and renewal. The ideas of restoration were not working, and a call for change could be heard from Africa to the Irish sea. Those in charge have had to explain their actions or inactions during the crisis years. What is it that brings the Catholic dream into a nightmare in roughly fifty years? Did we ever think that high ranking church clerics would choose past papal pronouncements over the lives of Catholics at risk for AIDS, particularly women and children? After all, popes are supposed to be pro-life. The answer can be found in the deliberations of Vatican II.

Lessons *not* Learned at Vatican II

There is no question that the council fathers wanted to teach Roman Catholics a new understanding of what it means to be church in the modern era.[3] Is there something wrong with the church? Is the church best thought of as the "People of God?" Does the church need to be brought up-to-date? These questions were probably on the mind of Bishop Emile de Smedt of Bruges, Belgium, when he delivered one of the great interventions of Vatican II. He claimed that the church of the 1950s smacked of clericalism, juridicism, and triumphalism, and that these defects were harming the church.[4] They were "isms" that had to go. The charges he leveled at "Holy Mother Church" did not sit well with his conservative brother bishops, but most of the clerics present praised his insights and delivery. The presentation hit home. We need to focus on the last term he used to critique the church, namely, "triumphalism," since it is key to understanding the dysfunctional behavior of Catholics—yesterday and today. Nothing is more important in this discussion of clerical misadventures and failures than probing the meaning of this term. Indeed, Bishop de Smedt was concerned about gold crosses, fancy rings, the white ermine cape the pope wears on special occasions, and the *sedia gestatoria*, that is, the 1960s version of the popemobile whereby the pontiff is carried from place to place by attendants while he was seated on a throne. But most of all, de Smedt objected to the way clerics "tried to lord it over others" in the church. These clerics considered themselves superior to the rest of Catholics, and that was not right; theirs was to be a servant ministry in the church. Brian Gleeson puts it this way: "Triumphalism places more importance on the prerogatives of authority stemming from valid institutional appointment, than on prayerful discernment . . . of the gifts of the Holy Spirit for ministry."[5]

Recall that when the papal birth control commission cast its final ballots on key propositions, only the votes of bishops and cardinals were counted and reported to the pope. Not even the votes of priests were part of the final report sent to the pope. That is Catholic culture. Elitism was alive and well in 1966 despite the new vision of "servant church" adopted by the council two years before.[6] The exaggerated belief that membership in the clerical state gives special access to the divine will leads us to the essential problem of triumphalism: there is an undervaluation of the majority of human beings in the church and an overemphasis on the divine character found in its principal leader: the Holy Father. The task of de Smedt and other council fathers was to strike a balance between the human and divine aspects of the church—the gifts of the Spirit and the gift of human creation.

The teaching on collegiality was, to some degree, an attempt to reign in the distortions of Vatican I about papal power and at the same time create an effective dialogue between today's bishop of Rome and the successors of the apostles. Cardinal Ottaviani represented the papist faction of the curia when he blurted out at the council one day that "the pope speaks alone" (*Il papa parla da solo*).[7] He does not need the college of bishops! This in no way expresses the teachings of Vatican II regarding the pope's role in the church. He is *not* the decider. All the bishops of the church in union with the pope are responsible and decide for the universal church. But when Paul VI let Ottaviani's views dominate discussion on birth control post–Vatican II, when he rejected the birth control commission's report, when he refused to call a synod to debate the two recommendations on birth control in 1967—yes, it was then that he let triumphalism back into the church. Collegiality was defanged by a small group of conservatives in the Roman Curia to the detriment of coherent theological discussion. The divine will was going to speak through the voices of a secretive group of conservative clerics who excluded those who disagreed with their point of view. God did not want their ideas, or so it seemed. Instead of a balanced approached to decision making, we get a process of theological gerrymandering—let's construct a system whereby the conservatives get the most votes! In the words of Cardinal Martini, the church needs change, major change. The current system, if left to its own devices, will come up with the wrong answers to important church problems repeatedly. The people of God will suffer. As we close this discussion, it is clear that several aspects of the church need change.

- By emphasizing their juridic power, popes have tended to see themselves on the defensive; they are the last wall of defense against heresy. In the future, popes must collaborate to solve complex problems because no one person has the totality of human experience nor all the answers.
- Leading church officials must avoid working with people who are too ideological and focused only on convincing others that they are right. Input from community groups can save the church.
- The future church, to avoid errors and celebrate the people of God theology, needs to involve laymen and women in major decisions. In the past we can see that the birth control commission got it right, but the pope ignored the laity in 1966 and that tendency has continued till this day.

WHAT'S THE ANSWER?

When an organization and its managers repeatedly make serious errors, the board of directors looks for new leadership. This of course does not describe how the Catholic Church functions. Church officials wait for the pope to die and then hope for changes to be made to improve things when a new pontiff is chosen. But when Pope Benedict XVI resigned in February 2013 at age eighty-five, citing health reasons and frailty, there emerged a window of opportunity that could not have been anticipated. At first, new Pope Francis looked like the right man for the job, but upon further review his resume does not describe a man hungry for change.

As cardinal of Buenos Aires, Argentina, Jorge Bergoglio never called on the pope publicly to allow the use of condoms to prevent the spread of

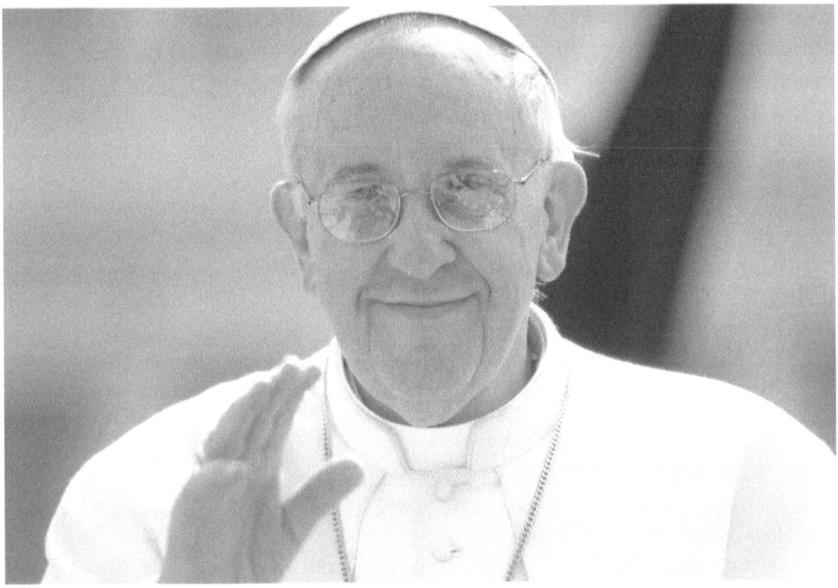

Image 12.1. Pope Francis, bishop of Rome.

AIDS. His recent actions affecting women religious in the United States fail to demonstrate a solid understanding of modern women professionals working in the church. At seventy-six he has a few good years left, and the best hope for change under his leadership would be a call to arms: a call for a council, Vatican III. The problems the church faces are too complex for one man and a group of cardinal consultants to resolve. His meeting in October 2013 with eight specially selected cardinals from around the world (only one from the Roman Curia) could be a first step in realizing the importance of a council.[8] Initially, the "Gang of 8" are to advise him on the governance of the universal church.[9] Down the road, other people need to be involved—clergy and laity—if the Catholic Church is to follow God's call of the new pope's patron saint, Francis of Assisi: "Go and rebuild my church which as you see is falling into ruin." One resolution that needs to pass quickly at any Vatican meeting this year is this: church officials must apologize to those families whose members died of AIDS needlessly. Benedict XVI should make that statement in public. Second, the plans to canonize John Paul II should be suspended. How could someone be declared a saint if he put thousands of Catholics at risk for getting AIDS by banning the use of condoms? That is not saintly behavior. Third, given what we know now about how *Humanae Vitae* came about, the pope and his consultants should call for a review of this teaching by an objective panel of Catholics who could render an unbiased report on the matter of artificial birth control.

In conducting research for this book I recall the words of a Filipino youth who was dying of AIDS. A social worker asked: "Why didn't you practice safe sex?" He replied: "I am a Catholic and my Church does not allow it." He was just following orders.

NOTES

1. Paul Moses, "Cardinal Martini's Last Interview," *Commonweal*, September 1, 2012.
2. *National Catholic Reporter*, April 14, 1995, 3.
3. *The Dogmatic Constitution of the Church* (*Lumen Gentium*) (Rome: 1964).
4. Avery Dulles, *Models of the Church* (New York: Doubleday/Image Books, 2002), 31.
5. Brian Gleeson, "Images, Understandings, and Models of the Church in History," *Australian E-Journal of Theology* 12 (2008).
6. Richard McBrien, "Vatican II Themes: The Church as Servant," *National Catholic Reporter*, August 1, 2011.
7. Bishop Remi De Roo, "Experiences of a Council Father," http://vatican2voice.org/92symp/deroo.htm (accessed June 25, 2013).
8. List of the eight cardinals: Pasinya (Congo), Gratias (India), Ossa (Chile), Bertello (Italy), Pell (Australia), Maradiaga (Honduras), O'Malley (Boston, MA), and Marx (Germany).
9. John Allen, "Pope Francis Taps Eight Cardinals to Lead Vatican Reform," *National Catholic Reporter*, April 13, 2013.

Appendix

CONDOMS ARE EFFECTIVE IN PREVENTING HIV/AIDS

Food and Drug Administration (FDA). Currently, FDA requires condom boxes and packets to state: "If used properly, latex condoms will help to reduce the risk of transmission of HIV infection (AIDS) and many other sexually transmitted diseases."

National Institutes of Health (NIH). According to the National Institutes of Health, condoms are impervious to the smallest viruses and only break or slip off 1 percent to 2 percent of the time. But surveys show many people don't use them properly or consistently.

James Trussell. He is director of Princeton University's Office of Population Research; he maintains that there is absolutely incontrovertible evidence that condoms reduce transmission of the most serious sexually transmitted disease, AIDS.

D. Halperin. "The time has come," *Lancet* (2004), 364: 1913. He states that the risk of HIV infection can be lowered by 80–90 percent with consistent and correct use of condoms.

Edward Green, Harvard University. "Condoms should be made available to everyone. The program should be Abstain, Be faithful, and use a Condom" (2009).

Centers for Disease Control, "Condoms and STDs," September 13, 2011; www.cdc.gov/condomeffectiveness/latex.htm (accessed June 1, 2012).

Bibliography

Allan, John. "Profile: New Pope, Jesuit Bergoglio, Was runner-Up in 2005 Conclave." *National Catholic Reporter*, March 3, 2013.

———. "Pope Francis Taps Eight Cardinals to Lead Vatican Reform." *National Catholic Reporter*, April 13, 2013.

Alsan, Marcella. "The Church & AIDS in Africa: Condoms & the Culture of Life." *Commonweal*, April 21, 2006.

Altman, Lawrence. "Blood Supply Called Free of AIDS." *New York Times*, August 1, 1985.

———. "Discoverers of AIDS and Cancer Viruses Win Nobel." *New York Times*, October 7, 2008.

Arie, Sophie. "Cardinal Says Condoms Could Help to Stop AIDS." *The Guardian (UK)*, February 1, 2005.

Bendavid, Eran, and Jayanta Bhattacharya. "The President's Emergency Plan for AIDS Relief in Africa: An Evaluation of Outcomes." *Annals of Internal Medicine* 150 (2009): 688–95.

Benedict XVI. *Light of the World* (A Conversation with Peter Seewald). San Francisco: Ignatius Press, 2010.

Blais, Mark, et al., "Personality and Personality Disorders." In *Massachusetts General Hospital Comprehensive Clinical Psychiatry*, 1st ed., edited by Theodore Stern et al. Philadelphia: Mosby Elsever, 2009.

Bongaarts, John, Francois Pelletier, and Patrick Gerland. "Global Trends in AIDS Mortality." Working Paper #16. Population Council. New York, 2009: 7.

———. "How many more AIDS deaths." *Lancet* 375 (2010): 103.

Brennan, Robert O., and David T. Durack. "Gay Compromise Syndrome." *Lancet* 318, no. 8259 (1981): 1338–39.

Butler, Declan. "Conclave Kindles Hope for Bioethical Reform." *Nature* 434 (April 21, 2005) 944.

Canadian Conference of Catholic Bishops. "Canadian Bishops' Statement on the Encyclical *Humanae Vitae*." Ottawa, Canada., September 27, 1968.

Centers for Disease Control (CDC). *Morbidity and Mortality Weekly Report* 50, no. 21 (2001).

———. "Condoms and STDs: Fact Sheet for Public Health Personnel." Atlanta, GA, U.S. Government Printing, 2008. February 8, 2010 last update. Also see: www.cdc.gov/condomeffectiveness/latex.htm (accessed June 5, 2013).

Chadwick, Henry. *The Early Church*. New York: Penquin, 1993.

Cichocki, Mark. "HIV around the World—South Africa." February 11, 2011. http://aids.about.com/od/clinicaltyrials/a /safrica_2.htm (accessed May 4, 2013).

Cockerham, William. *Sociology of Mental Disorder*, 8th ed. New York: Prentice Hall, 2011.

———. *Medical Sociology*. 12th edition. New York: Prentice Hall, 2012.

Congar, Ives. *My Journal of the Council*. Collegeville, MN: Liturgical Press, 2012.

Congregation for the Doctrine of the Faith. "Note regarding Certain Interpretations of 'Light of the World.'" Rome: Vatican Press, December 21, 2010.

Copson, Raymond. "CRS Issue Brief for Congress: AIDS in Africa." Catholic Relief Services, Washington, D.C., May 28, 2004.

Crawley, William. "The Pope Was Right about Condoms, Says Harvard HIV Expert." BBC News, March 29, 2009. www.bbc.co.uk/blogs/ni/2009/03/aids_expert_who_defended_the_p.html (accessed June 19, 2012).

De Roo, Remi. "Experiences of a Council Father." http://vatican2voice.org/92symp/deroo.htm (accessed June 25, 2013).

Dogmatic Constitution on the Church (*Lumen Gentium*), Second Vatican Council, November, 21, 1964.

Donadio, Rachel, and Laurie Goodstein. "After Condom Remarks, Vatican Confirms Shift." *New York Times*, November 23, 2010.

Dulles, Avery. *Models of the Church*. New York: Doubleday/Image Books, 2002.

Egan, Anthony. "The Pope on Condoms: Change or No Change?" *Thinking Faith: The Online Journal of the British Jesuits*, November 24, 2010. www.thinkingfaith.org/articles/20101124_2.htm (accessed April 17, 2012).

Ehlers, Fiona, et al. "Exhausted in the Vatican: The Final Battles of the Pope Benedict XVI." *Der Spiegel*, June 15, 2012.

Epstein, Helen. *The Invisible Cure*. New York: Farrar, Strauss, Giroux, 2007.

Fehring, Richard. "An Analysis of the Majority Report." *Life and Learning XIII* (2003), epublications.marquette.edu/nursing_fac/48/ (accessed June 9, 2012).

Fischl, M., D. Richman, et al. "The Efficacy of Azidothymidine (AZT) in the Treatment of Patients with AIDS." *New England Journal of Medicine* 317, no. 4 (1987): 185–91.

Fligstein, Neil, and Doug McAdam. "Toward a General Theory of Strategic Action Fields." *Sociological Theory* 29 (2011): 1–26.

Gibson, David. "The Catholic Church." *New York Times*, November 27, 2010.

Gleeson, Brian. "Images, Understandings, and Models of the Church in History." *Australian E-Journal of Theology* 12 (2008).

Goering, Laurie. "South African Bishop Bucks the Vatican." *Chicago Tribune*, November 4, 2005.

Goodstein, Laurie. "Catholics File Suits on Contraception Coverage." *New York Times*, May 21, 2012.
Gray, F. "Vatican to Rule on AIDS and Condoms." *CatholicHerald.co.uk*, April 28, 2006, 1.
Green, Edward. *Rethinking AIDS Prevention*. Westport, CT: Praeger, 2003.
———. "The Pope May Be Right." *Washington Post*, March 29, 2009.
———. *Broken Promises: How the AIDS Establishment Has Betrayed the Developing World*. Sausalito, CA: PoliPointPress, 2011.
Hockenos, Paul. "144 Theologians Confront Hierarchy." *National Catholic Reporter*, February 14, 2011.
Iliff, Laurence. "Mexican Bishop Backs Condom Use." *Dallas Morning News*, January 21, 2005.
Ingham, Robert. "No Praise for Pope from AIDS Campaigners." Agence France-Presse, April 4, 2005.
Ivereigh, Austen. "Pope on Condoms and AIDS." *America*, November 21, 2010.
———. "AIDS, Condoms, and the Suppression of Theological Truth." *America*, February 11, 2010.
———. "Towards a New Morality: Condoms and Church Teaching." *The Tablet*, November 27, 2010: 1–2.
———. "Rhonheimer: 'Benedict XVI Has Changed the Discourse on Aids and Condoms.'" *America*, December 7, 2010.
John Paul II. *Veritatis Splendor*. Rome: Vatican Press, 1993.
Johnson, Anne. "Regular Review: Heterosexual Transmission of Human Immunodeficiency Virus." *British Medical Journal 296* (1988): 1017–20.
Johnson, Dirk. "Ryan White Dies of AIDS at 18; His Struggle Helped Pierce Myths."*New York Times, April 9, 1990.*
Kaiser, Robert. *The Politics of Sex and Religion*. Kansas City, MO: Leaven Press, 1985.
Kaiser Family Foundation. "The Global HIV/AIDS Epidemic." *Fact Sheet*, June, 2001.
Kalbian, Aline. "Catholics and Contraception since 1968: Has Anything Really Changed?" *Louvain Studies* 36 (2012): 22–45.
Kelly, J. N. D. *The Oxford Dictionary of Popes*. New York: Oxford University Press, 1986.
Kimball, Charles. *When Religion Becomes Evil*. New York: HarperCollins, 2002.
König, Franz. "It Must be the Holy Spirit." *The Tablet* (December 21–28, 2002).
Kristof, Nicholas. "The Pope and AIDS." *New York Times*, May 8, 2005, A17.
Küng, Hans. *My Struggle for Freedom: Memoirs*. Grand Rapids, MI: Eerdmans, 2003.
———. "Church in Worst Credibility Crisis since the Reformation." *The Irish Times*, April 16, 2010.
Lancet. Editorial. "Redemption for the Pope?" *The Lancet* 373, no. 9669 (2009), 1054.
Liu, Cindy, et al. "Male Circumcision Significantly Reduces Prevalence and Load of Genital Anaerobic Bacteria." *mBio* 4, no. 2 (2013): e00076-13.DOI: 10.1128/mBio.00076-13.
Lockman, Shahin, Roger Shapiro, et al. "Response to Antiretroviral Therapy after a Single, Peripartum Dose of Nevirapine." *New England Journal of Medicine* 356 (2007): 135–47.

Loury, Erin. "Scientists Make Curing HIV a Priority." *Los Angeles Times*, July 23, 2012.

Martin, Douglas. "Cardinal John P. Foley, 76, Vatican Spokesman, Dies." *New York Times*, December 12, 2011.

Martin, William. *With God on Our Side: The Rise of the Religious Right in America*. New York: Broadway Books, 1997, 251.

McAdam, Doug. "Legacies of Anti-Americanism: A Sociological Perspective." In *Anti-Americanisms in World Politics*, edited by Peter Katzenstein and Robert Keohane, 251–69. Ithaca, NY: Cornell University Press, 2007.

McBrien, Richard. "Vatican II Themes: The Church as Servant." *National Catholic Reporter*, August 1, 2011.

McCarthy, John, and Mayer Zald. "Resource Mobilization and Social Movements." *American Journal of Sociology* 82 (1977): 1212–41.

McClory, Robert. *Turning Point*. New York: Crossroad, 1995.

McCormick, Richard. "'Humanae Vitae' 25 Years Later." *America*, July 17, 1993.

McGrath, Sophie. "In the Age of Dictators: Edith Stein and Pope Pius XI in Conversation." *Australian eJournal of Theology* 3 (August, 2004).

McNamara, Patrick, et al., "Dopaminergic Syndromes." *Sleep and Hypnosis* 4, no. 3 (2002): 119–31.

McNeil, Donald. "AIDS: A Price Break for Antiretroviral Drugs in 70 of the World's Poorest Countries." *New York Times*, May 23, 2011.

Moses, Paul. "Cardinal Martini's Last Interview." *Commonweal*, September 1, 2012.

Mumford, Stephen. "The Vatican's Role in the World Population Crisis: The Untold Story." *The Journal of Social, Political and Economic Studies* 20 (1995): 245–55.

National Catholic Register, 2007. www.ncregister.com/site/article/africas_catholic_explosion/ (accessed December 6, 2012).

O'Malley, John W. *What Happened at Vatican II*. Cambridge: Harvard University Press, 2008.

Oppenheimer, Mark. "A Cohort of Married Roman Catholic Priests, and More on the Way." *New York Times*, January 6, 2012.

O'Toole, James. *Creating the Good Life*. Emmaus, PA: Rodale, 2005.

Paul VI, *Humanae Vitae*. [Letter on Birth Control]. Rome: Vatican Press, 1968.

Pear, Robert. "AIDS Blood Test to Be Available in 2 to 6 Weeks." *New York Times*, March 3, 1985.

Piot, Peter. *No Time to Lose*. New York: Norton, 2012.

Piven, Frances Fox. "Can Power from Below Change the World." *American Sociological Review* 73 (2008): 1–14.

Pool, Robert. "Arcadia Doctor Recalls Consultation with Pope John Paul." *L.A. Times*, December 31, 2011.

Potts, Malcolm, Daniel Halperin, et al. "Reassessing HIV Prevention." *Science* 320 (2008): 749–50.

Prejean, Joseph, R. Song, et al. "Estimated HIV Incidence." *PLoS One* 6, no. 8 (2011): 24–36.

Pullella, Philip. "Vatican Broadens Case for Condoms to Fight AIDS" Reuters, November 24, 2010.

Ratzinger, Joseph. "Letter to the Bishops of the Catholic Church on the Pastoral Care of Homosexual Persons." Congregation for the Doctrine of the Faith, Rome, October 1, 1986.

Reese, Thomas. "Sex and the Fifth Commandment." *Washington Post*, November 22, 2010.

———. "On Sex Abuse." *America*, May 10, 2012.

Reinhold, Robert. "The Papal Visit; AIDS Issue at Fore as Pope Visits San Francisco Today." *New York Times*, Septmeber 17, 1987.

Rhodes, David, Lesley Ashton, et al. "Characterization of Long-Term Nonprogression." *Journal of Virology* 74, no. 22 (2000): 10581–88.

Rhonheimer, Martin. "The Truth about Condoms." *The Tablet*, July 10, 2004.

Riding, Alan. "Theologians in Europe Challenge Pope's Conservative Leadership." *New York Times*, July 14, 1989.

Rivera, John, and Mike Leary. "Pope John Paul II Dies." *Baltimore Sun*, April 3, 2005.

Rondy, John. "Catholic Church at the Crossroads in Milwaukee." Reuters, April 9, 2010. Also see www.reuters.com/article/idUSTRE6380S620100409 (accessed June 22, 2011).

Rynne, Xavier. *The Fourth Session*. London: Faber, Faber, 1966.

Scarisbrick, J. J. "An Historian's Reflections on Ybes Congar's Mon Journal de Concile." In *Yves Congar: Theologian of the Church*, edited by Gabriel Flynn. Louvain: Peeters Press, 2005.

Simon, V., D. D. Ho, and Karim Abdool. "HIV/AIDS Epidemiology, Pathogenesis, Prevention, and Treatment." *Lancet* 368 (2006): 489–504.

Simpson, Victor. "Pope Says Condoms Worsen HIV Problem." *Washington Post*, March 18, 2009.

Slevin, Gerald. "New Birth Control Commission Papers Reveal Vatican's Hand." *National Catholic Reporty*, March 23, 2011. http://ncronline.org/news/vatican/new-birth-control-commission-papers-reveal-vaticans-hand (accessed February 23, 2012).

Smith, William. "The Church." In *Aspects of Contemporary France*, edited by Sheila Perry. Paris: Action Press, 1989.

Srdan Matic et al. *HIV/AIDS in Europe*. Geneva: World Health Organization, 2006.

Steinfels, Peter. "Catholic Bishops Vote." *New York Times*, June 28, 1988.

Tobian, Aaron, David Serwadda et al. "Male Circumcision for the Prevention of HSV-2 and HPV Infections and Syphilis." *New England Journal of Medicine* 360 (2009): 1298–1309.

Trujillo, Alfonso. "Family Values versus Safe Sex." Paper of the Pontifical Council for the Family, December 1, 2003.

UNAIDS. "Global HIV/AIDS Response—Progress Report 2011." www.unaids.org/en/resources/publications/2011/name,644,en.asp (accessed June 9, 2012).

U.S. Catholic Bishops Administrative Board. "The Many Faces of AIDS: A Gospel Response." Washington, D.C., November 14, 1987.

U.S. Government Accountability Office. "Needle Exchange Programs," March 23, 1993.

Weiss, Gregory L., and Lynne E. Lonnquist. *The Sociology of Health, Healing, and Illness*, 7th edition. New York: Prentice Hall, 2012.

Wilde, Melissa J. "How Culture Mattered at Vatican II: Collegiality Trumps Authority in the Council's Social Movement Organizations." *American Sociological Review* 69, no. 4 (2004): 576–602.

Index

www.ingramcontent.com/pod-product-compliance
Ingram Content Group UK Ltd.
Pitfield, Milton Keynes, MK11 3LW, UK
UKHW041122071026
15587UKWH00009B/85

9 780739 17684